HAPPINESS LIES IN POSITIVE LIVING
BE POSITVE THINK POSITIVE LIVE POSITIVE

BY

BALDEV BHATIA

I0425712

ABOUT THE BOOK

INTRODUCTION

Happiness Lies in Positive Living.

Be Positive Think Positive Live Positive

What do we think about Positivity? The feeling of positivity is within us. It is said that positive living is purely an internal matter. It has nothing to do with our external circumstances. There is something positive within us who keep us happy and there is something negative within us which keep you unhappy. Happy living through positivity is nothing more than that of living a normal life free from undue pressures, problems and tensions. If we want to live a happy life then we need to get rid of the negativity within us which makes us unhappy. Negative approach always complicates the problems and increases unhappiness? Most of us do the fatal mistake of looking outwards for happiness rather than looking inwards. Be positive, be strong, be bold and be courageous every day. Even if we are having a bad day, think of some good things that may come our way, either later that day, tomorrow, next week, month, or year. When everything seems to be beyond our control, it's almost too easy for us to slip into the grasp of negativity. To avoid negativity we must strive to abolish this sort of thinking through the power of thinking positively. The Art of Positive Living is not a complicated kind of art difficult to learn rather a simple art of positive thinking, living well, eating well, thinking well and feeling well.

What we need to do is just to tune up our mind to enjoy every moment of life and let the positive happiness follow us. This is something that needs to be looked into thoroughly. We need to focus on the positive aspects lives, rather than on the negative setbacks. We must remember that positive living is the reward of positive thinking. We ought to remember, only the positive thinking can bring happiness in our lives. If we cannot think positively, you cannot live happily. Be our own teacher or adviser we ought to look everything with a positive angle. Let us find something good even in most critical moments of our life and let us make positive thinking the basis of our happy living. It's a matter of thought that fools worry about the circumstances on which they have no control. Why worry when we cannot change the climate, rather enjoy it whether it's hot, humid, cold, cloudy, foggy or snowy. Let us all keep our internal weather mind body and soul pleasant all the time. A sound and positive happiness is all around. It's not far away from us. If we do not want to live happy, it's up to us. It's our own choice. We must not blame others, nor should we blame our fate or external circumstances. Another thing is that feeling confident affects the way we perceive our situations and how we decide to manage them.

Think that by being more optimistic we alter our approaches to situations and take on them in a healthier manner; we think of alternatives and act according to better outcomes. If we think positive it will be positive. It does not say to stick our heads in the soil; rather it says to think positive. Interestingly it does not say feel positive it says think positive and that is the real meaning to remain happy. Happiness does not come alone, it adds our minds body and soul to remain in constant touch with each other. We have to remove negative thoughts and create and atmosphere to be happy in our lives. There are many fear factors that are reasoning us to be unhappy and the main reason being that our heart and our feelings which are more susceptible to fear and worry then the mind. Of course we do the worrying in our minds but it is our emotions that are worried not our brains. When the heart senses the possibility of loss it can start panicking and then uses the mind to worry and many times tries to manipulate the brain in dealing with the fear. The heart desires something and gets excited about it and then it manipulates the mind to assure that it will get it. Although the brain can control the emotions and knowledge precedes all, however when it comes to response time the brain is slower than the emotions. That is which explains why we say or do things and then regret them. Our objective in life should be to train ourselves to wait for the brain to show up before we say or do anything. Fear usually comes from the emotions and thinking positive is something the brain is capable of doing. It would be very hard to tell someone who is worried to feel positive. But if you tell them to think positive that is something even a worried person can do. We need to use our mind to think positive, to think of a positive outcome. Thinking positive brings positive results in its wake; when you react in a positive way to a negative situation you usually get positive in return. Positive mental attitude is effective in many ways. There are limits to the effectiveness of positive thinking. It is not always enough to change deeply entrenched irrational core beliefs about self, others and the world. When someone does something to us do we think about it in a positive way or in a negative way? Do we try to assume that the person who is not treating us the way we should be treated is themselves in pain and needs our love or do we assume that they just don't like us and therefore we need to respond back in kind? It is therefore a must for us to learn understand and remember that we need to be positive and think positive in the interest of our happy living.

SD /-

(BALDEV BHATIA)

   AUTHOR   **MAY 13TH 2016**

HAPPINESS LIES IN POSITIVE LIVING
BE POSITVE THINK POSITIVE LIVE POSITIVE
PREFACE

Author Baldev Bhatia shares with millions of curious readers the 'real knowledge' by letting them know more about themselves in detail through their born qualities along with the help of the positive qualities possessed by them and to ward off the negativity in them and also get to know the ways as how to live happily. The worries adopted by them, the negative forces influencing them, need to be discarded for a positive and happy living.A thought of penning down the wonders of the mystic manuscript of the negative forces influencing the masses with their thoughts has lured the author cum astrologer to bring to the millions of readers the 'real knowledge' by letting them know more about themselves in detail with the help of astrological science to know more about their Zodiac Signs, their habits, characteristics; appearances; their personality; profession, career; business, finances, their match with other zodiac signs; romance, marriage, weakness their health and disease and finally the negative forces possessed by them and to ward of this negativity factor with the guidance of this manuscript charming them to become more positive so that they can lead a happy life.This Microscopy of Positive Living is based on the practical experience of the author who has meet several thousand people having negativity in their personal lives and those leading a miserable life totally being depressed and dejected. The main purpose of writing this manuscript is to impart the basic knowledge of how to become bold, strong, courageous, and how to throw away the negative forces in them. This manuscript reveals a whole lot of information when one is in search for the truths of a positive attitude. With this the author shares his experience with his readers. His published books "Microscopy of Astrology", Microscopy of Numerology", Microscopy of Remedies also guides his readers to achieve their personal goals with ease and assist them to overcome all the problems, crises, and the unforeseen negatives forces, in their lives so as to avoid getting disheartened or depressed. This book goes to reveal, ascertaining the real facts of life and the destiny as to what is stored for each and every reader in his or her future. Various chapters have been covered and maximum emphasis have been paid to cover the subjects pertaining to the significance of positivity by reading different charts; different Zodiac signs, planets and their placements in different houses and signs; affliction of planets with the interpretation of the major period and the meaning of the birth signs and also the zodiac compatibility of the individual birth signs.

Author and Astrologer Baldev Bhatia have put his entire life experience in promoting positivity among his clients through this mystic science of Astrology. He has done so in order to serve millions of curious readers with a good intension of imparting them the basic knowledge of how to become a positive person in life. The author-cum astrologer has been associated with general public for the past 45 years and has been practicing phycology and pubic healing. His intension is also to guide the readers to achieve their personal goals with ease and would assist them to overcome all the problems, crises, speed breakers and the unforeseen negatives forces, in their lives as not to get disheartened or depressed in their lives.The Author's main object and message, through this manuscript to his readers is to spread, Peace, Love happiness to the entire world and tries to guide his readers to ward off negativity, depression, dejection and hatred among them. He has done his best to reveal to his readers to attain positivity in way or manner irrespective of all the hardships and to attain a path of glory by getting away from their weakness of negative thinking and discarding forever the depression dejection by way of adopting a positive attitude to be bold to be strong and to be courageous, through which they can lead a positive happy and prosperous life.

This book also intends to guide the readers to achieve their personal goals with ease that would assist them to overcome all the problems, crises, speed breakers and the unforeseen negatives forces, in their lives, as not to get worried or disheartened or depressed in their lives if the influence of the Transiting Planets is weak, guesting depressing, unfavorable and disappointing. This books goes to emphasis that if the influence is good, it brings good or positive changes or events in life. But negative influence gives undesired results. One needs to understand that no matter what aspect a transiting planet makes to natal planets, the individual need to hold on his nerves to be bold to be strong and to be positive in life whatever be the circumstances governing his future and the positive energy that is already stored in him. . The chapters in the book are very useful, purposeful, and a pin point to the service of mankind. He wishes success for all his readers. The author would definitely like to express my sincere thanks to Ms. Alpa Shah Director, Travel Company of UK, for helping and encouraging him to pen down this book in the interest of depressed and dejected and the so called Negative persons of this universe. The author is also grateful and thankful to Publishers for publishing this book

Dated: May 13th 2016   **BALDEV BHATIA**
AUTHOR

HAPPINESS LIES IN POSITIVE LIVING
BE POSITVE THINK POSITIVE LIVE POSITIVE
ABOUT THE AUTHOR

Astrology has stood the test of times ever since it revealed the Mystery and the Mastery of the ancient wisdom of forecasting the influence of the stars on human bodies. The author Baldev Bhatia a renowned and world famous Astrologer has penned several simple books on Astrology-this mysterious subject that reveals the true perception of knowing oneself through the art of prediction.

Professionally the author has put his entire life experience in promoting Astrology in various fields with a view to serve the millions of curious readers of this mystic science with the intension of imparting them the real knowledge of Astrology through various marvelous scriptures.

The Astrologer has been associated with Astrology for the past 45 years and has been practicing Astrology in various forms.

The Author-cum Astrologer has been in touch with general public throughout his life and has been practicing phycology and pubic healing.

His intension is to guide his readers to achieve their personal goals with ease that would assist them to overcome all the problems, crises, speed breakers and the unforeseen negatives forces, in their lives so as not to get disheartened or depressed in their lives and finally lead a happy life and peaceful life, after going through this manuscript of "Microscopy of Positive Living". More over Mr. Baldev Bhatia the Author is an established writer himself with a sound reputation of being a good Astrologer has put his valuable life experience in promoting positivity among his clients. The author also shares with millions of curious readers the 'real knowledge' by letting them know more about themselves in detail and also about their in born positive qualities, possessed by them and guides them to ward off the negativity in them, by getting to know as how to lead an happy and powerful life., without caring for the worries troubling them, the negative forces influencing them, which needs to be discarded forever, for a positive and happy living if the influence of the Planets happens to be unfavorable, negative and disheartening.

The main object of writing this manuscript is to impart the basic knowledge of how to become positive, bold, strong, courageous, and how to throw away the negative forces and become a happy person in life.

The author also shares the valuable experience of his life with his readers through his valuable and helpful book. His published books "Microscopy of Astrology", Microscopy of Numerology", Microscopy of Remedies, Microscopy of Happy Living guide his readers to achieve their personal goals with ease and assists them to overcome all the problems, crises, and the unforeseen negatives forces, in their lives gracefully which guides them not get disheartened or depressed at any stage of life irrespective of all the odds and negative forces troubling them. His readers have gained good experience going through his useful and purposeful books. His books have made his readers to feel secure, sound and have also encouraged them to face their destiny with immense strength and have also given them the power to face the challenges of this universe with utter confidence zeal and power.The author Baldev Bhatia leads way to happiness, success, positivity and advices his people suffering from depression and negativity in their personal lives to wake up and lead a positive and happy. After meeting hundreds and hundreds of depressed dejected disappointed and unhappy people from all over the world and people from all walks of life and he being a highly experienced Astrologer and Consultant in Astrology and Numerology felt it necessary to write books on

Happiness, Love, Peace which could guides his readers to ward of their depression, dejection, hatred and negativity in their lives.His books have also revealed to his readers to attain positivizes in their lives so that they could easily achieve their path of glory and reach to be a positive and happy person and also be a brave strong and courageous human being. His books have given gracefully accepted by the people worldwide. His books have helped the masses to achieve and lead a life full of positivity, boldness, strength, courage happiness and have generated confidence in depressed and dejected people. His books have helped his clients and readers to lead a good, peaceful and happy life. His books have been very different as they guide and help the readers to strengthen their will power and confidence which the readers have lost in today's world. In order to encourage his readers and to help them, in all walks of life the esteem Author finally decided to manuscript the following books in the interest and happiness of the universal world.

1.   **Microscopy of Astrology**

2.   **Microscopy of Numerology**

3.   **Microscopy of Remedies**

4.   **Microscopy of Happy Living**

All published by Partridge India Put Ltd

(A Penguin Publishing Company)

He finally wishes his readers all the success happiness and prosperity. He always praises God and prayers Him with the following words.

"May the Heavens Shower Peace Prosperity and Happiness to All"

"GOD BLESS YOU"

"THANKS FOR READING "

BALDEV BHATIA

May 16th 2016

HAPPINESS LIES IN POSITIVE LIVING
BE POSITVE THINK POSITIVE LIVE POSITIVE

INDEX

'

HAPPINESS LIES IN POSITIVE LIVING

BE POSITVE THINK POSITIVE LIVE POSITIVE

CHAPTER ONE

ANALYZING POSITIVITY

KNOW ABOUT YOURSELF AND YOUR POSITIVITY THROUGH

SIGNIFICANCE OF DIFFERENT ZODIAC SIGNS

ARIES **(21st March –19th April)**

Your Ruling Planet   **Mars**

Your Sign   **Fiery**

Born in Sign   **Movable**

CHARACTERISTIC

Your shall have round eyes, shall be quite talkative and urguementive. Short tempered, angry and bilious in nature. Tend to be the eldest of of the children, shall be popular, stingy and unsteady in behavior, moment of arms, hands and fingers are frequently seen while in conversation with others. Full of vigor, honored by the government, sparingly eating habits and shall have few children in life.

Appearance:

A good physique with large bones. Your features and your teeth tend to be good and even you are of medium height and you tend to develop into a unique punchy personality.

Personality:

You possess forceful, courageous, enterprising and industrious instincts. You refuse to give up until and unless you have not achieved your targets. Winning or losing is not very important to you, giving a good effort and showing a good account of your abilities is quite something where you are more cautious about. In your approach and speech you are quite confident even though you are not equipped with much knowledge of that subject. You are straightforward in your speech and would often not; hesitate in calling a thief a thief.

Calling a thief a thief doesn't always make you popular and even though you're fully aware of this, you really won't care much about others feeling and shall stick to your comments. You neither like pressures being forced upon you nor would like subordination, but would rather wish to be free in thoughts and action, and would love, free style of functioning. You are best suited for guiding, controlling and governing others. You can be very self-assertive, and well equipped to deal with any situation or emergency when the situation demands. You tend to be over optimistic and too impulsive and later regret your actions or inaction and at times overshoot the mark or over trade in business. Because of your impulsiveness you don't hesitate to get into an argument or pick up a quarrel over petty things .You are not the kind of person who would look before you leap, consistency is also not your virtue. Even if you happen to occupy a humble or subordinate position you will try to be at the head of some branch of your work or assignment. Whether in profession or business you will cross all barriers and speed breakers to attain success.

Profession and Career

You are best suited for a career connected with Metals, Engineering, Metallurgy, Surgery and you often tend to become good trade union leaders. Explorers, Explosives, Teachers, Self-Employed Professionals or the business people. Dealers of firearms, Dentists, Mechanics, and Sportsmen are the other fields where you would excel well.

Business and Finances

Though you have a good head for business but when it comes to making investments or tying up new deals, your become quite impulsive and rash. With the result your profits are cut off or minimized, but your financial position remain quite stable.

As you're prone to overrating your own judgment, it is you're over confidence, which combines with your impulsiveness that cuts off or reduces your profits. However, you're able to pull back yourself from major disasters and you do not remain a debtor for long.

You Match with   Aries, Leo Scorpions and Sagittarius

Romance and Marriage

You warm hearted nature will provide you with excellent chance for love and romance. But you must restrain yourself from being rash and impulsive. You expect your loved ones to share your thoughts and to respond to your moods in all situations. Your love life is quite stylish, and your living is luxurious. Romance and Love means a lot to you and you not hesitate in keeping everything aside until you get your desires fulfilled.

YOUR WEAKNESS

You will be such a bad liar that others can immediately see through you. But however selfish you may be, you will feel the sense of your selfishness if pointed out to you and you will readily accept the fact. Since you are a quick-witted, restless character, you may find it too difficult to be patient in any situation, which you do not like. You will put up with adverse conditions only as long as you are confident about it and you will eventually bring about the changes as per your desire and wishes even though you may have to take unnecessary risks in achieving your goals. Bravery and disregard for danger are inheritance in you.

You have the capacity to rapidly grasp the essential of a situation, but you shall also have its drawbacks, for not in seeing the whole shape of a problem, they might appear to be resulting in an argument, and leading to give an offence .You may be quick-tempered, but will be at your worst, extremely selfish, and demanding if such an occasion arises.

Health and Disease

The body parts ruled by your sign are muscles, head, and the eyes, and the face. You are quite prone to headaches, head injuries, brain disorders, and burns, are the other positive pointers. Minor accidents are also not ruled out.

You are person who could be recognized by a fine facial bone structure with a shining healthy head of hair. Definitely you are not weak people. You are mostly in a hurry and often do not get time to eat properly, with the result you tend to suffer from stomach ailments because low diet. At times you are subject to blood pressure, heart-related problems, and headaches including sinus and migraines.

As most conditions apply, plenty of water is essential for your body and you should take regular diet and complete rest, whenever excess stress or strain is promulgated.

Lucky Day   **Tuesday**

Lucky Colors   **Red and white.**

Lucky Stones   **Red Coral, Ruby, Garnet Blood Stone.**

Lucky Numbers 9, 18, 27, 36, 45, 54, 63 and 7

HAPPINESS LIES IN POSITIVE LIVING
BE POSITVE THINK POSITIVE LIVE POSITIVE
CHAPTER TWO
ZODIAC SIGNS

TAURUS (20th April -20th May)

Your Ruling Planet   Venus

Your Sign   Earth

Born in Sign   Fixed

CHARACTERISTIC

Ruled by Venus, the planet of love, you are good and sympathetic, caring and loyal. It is often said that you are a good lover of beauty. Your sense of preservation is far developed. Your strong will power generally carries you to great heights even when you are under severe stress and strain conditions. You have tendency to put on weight even though you are strong and well built. You love to have good food and prefer to take high fat diet and enjoy living in comfortable surroundings. At times when you tend to be lazy, and unwilling to do the job or work assigned to you, with the result that you loss the fruitful gains that are stored for you.

You're concerned with gaining material wealth and status and you make a sincere effort in achieving them. You have excellent business sense, the ability to make money. You are generous in entertaining your friends, and you enjoy the company of friends much more than the others do. You shall feel happier living in the big cities rather than in small towns.

Appearance

You are well built and hefty and you tend to put on weight easily. Your eyes are attractive and your body appearance resembles to a bull. Your lips are well shaped and your skin is soft and glowing. Your movements are quite graceful and well matched. You have broad face stout shoulders with big belly.

Personality

You are a popular learned and sensuous personality. You are practical, persevering and you have good powers of endurance. You often make faithful and loyal friends. You are very careful about your personal comforts and money matters. You are unreasonably stubborn at times, and you lose other people' sympathy in process. You have great power of endurance and patience, but when provoked to anger, your become wild, volatile and would not mind using abusive language. You have a strong will power and are quite conservative in your thoughts and actions.

You are bit slow but steady in actions .You would not to waste surplus energy and talent. You would plodder around a subject for pretty long till you are sure about it. You would only than act fast and wisely and see to it, that the concerned matters go to your advantage and favor .You are fond of ease, comforts and luxuries. You become worldly and take pleasure in the good things of life.

Profession and Careers

You would have a good taste for Arts, Music, Theatre, and Cinema .You would also make good singers, dancers, and art and jewelry dealers. Writers, models, actors are the other fields where you excel pretty well. Architects, financiers, bankers, are optional field, which fancy you.

Business and Finances

You make excellent business people and financiers and are known as the money zone of the zodiac. You manage to find opportunities to increase your profits or expand your business where others see none. You also tend to instinctively find above average avenues of investment. The best deals that you strike are generally those connected with land or property. You work happily as Florist, in Livestock or Poultry industry or are often seen as heads of Super Markets and wholesale food industrialist.

You Match with

Taurus, Gemini Virgo, Capricorn, and Aquarius.

Romance and Marriage

Since Venus, which powers you with physical charm, governs you happen to become a good humorist, thus radiating warmth and vitality around you. You are amorous by nature and you find it difficult to restrain the affections one bestowed upon you. You are also easily influenced by the attraction of the opposite sex. You make friends easily and are quite popular with fairer sex. Its a different matter that your romance begins only after you have satisfied yourself or have observed that your partner has the qualities that appeal to you. You are emotionally attached to their spouse once married, you look for unshakable stability. Your patience in personal relationships ensures you with stability and smoothness. You generally full fill your duties and obligations towards your loved ones.

Health and Disease

Though you are a good eater of delicious foods you would at the same time. Love to exercise and help your self in maintaining good health. Your sign rules, tongue and ears, the neck, throat, vocal chords, tonsils, thyroid gland, chin, lower jaw .You are prone to colds, coughs, sore throats, tonsillitis, obesity, blood pressure and constipation.

YOUR WEAKNESS

You can easily be misled by emotions and affections. You tend to be quite jealous and sentimental with regards to the matter of sex. You are dominating and obstinate with the result you almost lose the ground, which you have gained during your interaction with opposite sex. But once you find that everything around you is smooth and the grass is green and lovely you plunge head long to build a happy home and would like to create a world of your own nature.

Lucky Day	**Friday**
Lucky Colors	**Blue and violet**
Lucky Stones	**Diamond, white zircon.**
Lucky Numbers	**6, 15, 24, 33, 42 and 51**

HAPPINESS LIES IN POSITIVE LIVING
BE POSITVE THINK POSITIVE LIVE POSITIVE
CHAPTER THREE
ZODIAC SIGNS

GEMINI   21st May to 20th June

Your Ruling Planet   MERCURY

Your Sign   AIR

Born in Sign   Movable

CHARACTERISTIC

You are an airy sign you live mostly in the mind. You will be carefree, joyous and reluctant. Your mind will be strong and positive and strong. You are often versatile. Restless and inclined to changes and make improvements whenever there is necessity. You also appreciate traveling in search of adventure and amusement. Your enjoyment of the use of words enhances your ability to converse. You are quick, perceptive, clever, playful and imaginative, and you express yourself to feel alive. You feel fresh when you can move around mentally and physically unrestricted. Your ability to bluff your way out of tight corners is phenomenal, and you will always be on the go. You will be doing more than one thing at a time. This dual phenomenon is an important part of your nature. You need plenty of variety and change. You can very easily become bored, and your answer to drop whatever is boring to you is quite certain and to take, the next job in hand is one of your charactericts. You should be careful not to overstrain your sensitive nervous system, which can break down under pressure. You enjoy mental recreation, but you also appreciate traveling in search of adventure and amusement. If you're not interested in something, you can be indifferent to your liking and friendship. You love to be in company and attempt a whole variety of things simultaneously.

Appearance

Describing the Gemini is as mercurial is right on the money, since Gemini is ruled by the Planet Mercury. Moving, restless, seeking, learning -- Gemini is constant motion, a torrent of wind which is in keeping with this sign's element of Air. The Twins are highly intellectual and won't hesitate to play mind games with a lover, mere child's play to them. They are also great communicators, so get ready to hear everything from pithy remarks to impassioned pleas. Inventive, quick-witted and fun, the Twins will jump around from one lover to the next until they find one which is almost as smart as they are and able to keep up in this high-spirited race. The reward for those who can lasso a Gemini is a free-spirited lover who shines at parties but is also a devil in the bedroom.

Personality

A fine bone structure and movements that are light often set you apart from others and make you good dancers as well. Your facial expressions are usually baby like in their transparency. Quick to smile, with ears that are a bit larger than normal, your physique tends to remain slim even when your food intake begins to cross the limits .The Gemini is always right and never changes his mind - until the next time the argument comes around, when he will take a totally different stand, and deny ever having given vent to his earlier opinions.

This is infuriating for his opponents in argument, especially as he has a considerable talent for dialogue - and a tendency to know a very little about a very great number of things, and to master this knowledge skillfully as to seem well informed. His ability to bluff his way out of tight corners is phenomenal. There then, are his worst faults - inconsistency and superficiality. Little wonder, perhaps, that the world's most popular journalists in newspaper, radio, and television are

Gemini's. For again, they have an insistent urge to communicate.

Profession and Career

You would make good writers, radio and TV producers or anchor people, lecturers, linguists, teachers, travel agents, sales people.

Business and Finances

Like air, you feel fresh when you can move around mentally and physically unrestricted. But when traveling, you're likely to take along beepers, mobile phones, laptop computers, portable radios and televisions, and remote controls. You like being busy, juggling two or more things at once. Boredom, censure or repression could make you impatient, restless, anxious, snappish, sarcastic, gossipy, cynical or nervously exhausted

You Match with   Leo Gemini, Libra and Aquarius

Romance and Marriage

A love affair with a Gemini requires great stamina; so start doing those push-ups now! The Twins are both fun and funny and love to laugh, play and romp. They are possessed of a very active mind, which can sometimes lead to a short attention span. The best way to keep the

Twins around, and aroused, is through mental stimulation. A razor-sharp and imaginative lover is a godsend to the terrific Twins. This sign also values adventure and travel, so a certain footloose and fancy free-ness will help this romance bloom.

The duality of the Twins allows them to see both sides of an issue, so in times of stress, they are much likelier to be a lover than a fighter. They will also feel especially connected to those who can help them feel, since they spend so much of their time thinking. It's true that your attentions tend to stray even after marriage but it's also true that responsibilities gradually change your attitude and force you into being steady wives and husbands. And yet, you love your home and family and want the best for them. Resolving contradictions where you want to remain free and yet have a good family life are essential for you.

YOUR WEAKNESS

Someone who can roll with the punches and keep smiling in the face of a multi-faceted onslaught is priceless to the hyperactive Twins. It's an added plus if that person is smart, fun, a good friend and a great sport. Gemini's need someone who can be attentive to them and who will naturally enjoy their sparkle and wit. They also prefer a strong partner who is not necessarily as smart as they are but who can pick them up, emotionally, when necessary. If the Twins can make a marvelous mental match, life will be a dream. The Gemini lover is easygoing and caring, yet daring and a ball of fire at the right moments. Mental fireworks are high on their agenda, their own as well as those they can make with another. Only those with plenty of punch need apply for this celestial light show! The Gemini is always right and never changes his mind - until the next time the argument comes around, when he will take a totally different stand, and deny ever having given vent to his earlier opinions. This is infuriating for his opponents in argument, especially as he has a considerable talent for dialogue - and a tendency to know a very little about a very great number of things, and to master this knowledge skillfully as to seem well informed. His ability to bluff his way out of tight corners is phenomenal. There, then, are his worst faults - inconsistency and superficiality. Little wonder, perhaps, that the world's most popular journalists in newspaper, radio, and television are Gemini's. For again, they have an insistent urge to communicate.

Health and Disease

You suffer from allergies, asthma and frequent colds and flu. The skin, hair, veins as well as throat, kidneys and lumbar region of Gemini's get easily affected.

Lucky Day	**Wednesday**
Lucky Color	**Yellow**
Lucky Stone s	**Yellow Carnelian Agate)**
Lucky Numbers	**3, 12, 21, 30, 48, 57**

HAPPINESS LIES IN POSITIVE LIVING
BE POSITVE THINK POSITIVE LIVE POSITIVE
CHAPTER FOUR
ZODIAC SIGNS

CANCER   (22nd June-22nd July)

Your Ruling Planet	**Moon**
Your sign	**Water**
Born in Sign	**Movable**

CHARACTERISTIC

You are changeable, moody, restless and sensitive. You are emotional, tenacious, honest, intelligent, industrious, and miserly. Though proud, talkative, quite independent in your feelings, you are more attached to your home and family.

Physical Appearance

Usually of medium height, your build is sturdy and stocky. Your complexion is generally smooth and free from pimples and blemishes. Most of you have a strong, muscular physique with largish bones. Even symmetrical teeth and a wide mouth.

Personality

Your sign of water makes your nature moody. You tend to keep your emotions hidden in the innermost of your heart. This watery sign also bestows the powers of intuition. You possess strong pioneering instincts and are generally enterprising and industrious. In crunch situations, you are forceful a courageous and refuse to give up until you have achieved your targets or at least put in your best. Like a true sportsperson, you like to play for the challenge and enjoyment and at one level, winning or losing is not so important, what matters more to you is giving a good account of yourself. You are sensitive and take a fancy to anything, which comes new to you. In your speech and approach, you are direct and forthright. You are very particular about having good food. You're generally easy to get along with.

Your bad eating habits may often lead you to bad health. You don't like pressures being on you and value an easy going, free style of functioning. You tend to be too impulsive and later regret your actions or inaction. You're often also too outspoken and undiplomatic.

Profession and Career

Being hard working and industrious, you are successful in your own profession and business. You often reach high position in life. You generally make good Engineers, Explorers, Metal Workers, Dentists,

Surgeons, Mechanics, Self-employed Professionals or Business People. You do well in teaching, writing, painting, advertising, and selling things and also in trade and commerce, particularly, imports and exports.

Business and Finance

Although you have a good head for business and your financial position is usually stable, you're prone to overrating your own judgment, especially when it comes to making investments or tying up new deals. It's your impulsive nature and you're over confidence, which combine to cut it to your profits. Generally, however, you're able to pull back from major disasters and the saving grace is that you'll never remain a debtor. You are highly ambitious when it comes to amassing wealth, but you have to climb an uphill task in achieving the same. Wealth often eludes you even when you inherit your parental property or wealth. You should avoid betting, speculation and horseracing, as you are more likely to lose, rather than gain.

You Match with

Cancer, Leo, Scorpio, Sagittarius and Pisces

Romance and Marriage

You will enjoy your family life. Home and family are of great importance to you and will manage to keep your spouse quite happy and gay. You have a good style of admiration and you indulge in light flirtations. Many of you, despite your deep-seated desire to set up a home, are averse to marriage.

Part of the reason for this is that you are unable to disclose your inmost emotions and feelings even when your heart beats in tune to a strong love tone. Often, you tend to be attracted to an opposite number. Love means a lot to you and you're generally willing to put everything else aside until it fulfills your desires. Warm and loving, you often shower your through various means which includes paying profuse compliments, showering gifts, making stylish dates. Whether you're a male or a female you are usually very frank and forthright and you like to make it clear at the outset itself whether you're simply flirting or whether you are serious in your love and romantic affairs.

HEALTH AND DISEASE

You are likely to suffer from water borne diseases, comprising of gastric trouble, inflammatory troubles of liver, minor boils and infection in stomach. At times mental depression and excitement. Diabetes is one factor, where you need to be beware of.

YOUR WEAKNESS

You are lustful, drunkard and fickle minded. You become irritable and your crooked eyes speak of your lust and greed at several occasions.

Lucky Colors   **Green, mauve, mountain blue.**

Lucky Stones   **Emerald, pearl, cat's eye.**

Your Lucky Numbers   **2, 11, 20 29,**

HAPPINESS LIES IN POSITIVE LIVING
BE POSITVE THINK POSITIVE LIVE POSITIVE
CHAPTER FIVE
ZODIAC SIGNS

LEO **(23rd July-22nd August)**

Your **Planetary Ruler** **Sun**

Your Element **Fire**

Born in Sign **Fixed**

CHARACTERISTIC

You are extremely sympathetic, generous, honest, straightforward and authoritative. You are honest, frank, and outspoken. You are enterprising and like to command. In fact, your strongest instinct is to rule and command. You love authority. You are quite proud and lucky in money matters. You possess a strong will power and you achieve your objectives in spite of the difficulties or obstacles that come in your way. You are enterprising, soft but outspoken helpful and righteous personality. You are sincere, reputed, independent, impatient bold, generous and a respectable person. A traveler, obstinate and a happy go lucky person. You are affectionate, enthusiastic, cheerful, and optimistic whom, bring sunshine into other lives.

Appearance

You are tall, physically strong, and attractive and have a fair complexion. You have broad shoulders and have beautiful eyes with abundant energy. Your constitution is generally robust; you appear to have fashioned round face with model looks.

Personality

You are inclined to quick anger. Success comes to you only after much struggle. You would remain devoted to your parents. Your wife would be virtuous and happy lady.

Physically, you are strong and if you happen to fall ill, you will recover soon. You are both courageous and valorous. You never want to giveaway. You shun inferior jobs and are fond of a life of luxury works and jobs. You have a strong desire to travel, and you prefer to have an aristocratic society.

Professions and Career

The career best suited for you are Civil Services, Finance, Politics, Armed Forces, Business of Commanding Nature, You are quite courteous, diplomatic and do well in all professions where you may have to deal with dignified people .You are not generally good in dealing with masses or where laborers are involved. Your life starts to boom and you have the tendency to earn money at much younger age.

Business and Finances

You are magnanimous and are, therefore, unable to save in proportion to your income. Business partnerships lead to litigation, which should be settled out of court. There is a danger of part of your property being destroyed by fire. In financial matters, you may not get a square deal from your brothers and sisters, and this may even lead to litigation.

You Match With   Aries, Leo, Sagittarius and Gemini.

Romance and Marriage

You love steadfastly, and usually get married fairly early. However, being stubborn, you do not have a smooth relationship with your partner. You want to be overbearing, and unless the partner is submissive and docile, this leads to frequent clashes.

YOUR WEAKNESS

You tend to have a lot of ego and pride, and you have a certain amount of vanity by which you are easily ruffled. Your inimical feelings continue for a long time. You are pompous and prefer to show off your splendor on many occasions. You at times get suspicious, even when there is no substantial cause. You are inclined towards betting, gambling speculation, and games of chance. The greed of becoming rich at one go often attracts you.

HEALTH AND DISEASE

The heart and the aorta, upper back, spleen and the spinal chord form your major vulnerable health areas and can result in heart diseases, back problems, or spinal meningitis. Your sign rules the heart and back, and your tendency to drive yourself hard, often puts them under pressure. The pressure increases because you enjoy good food and are prone to be overweight. For good health, you've got to respect your body's needs.

Lucky Days   **Sundays**

Lucky Color   **Red, orange, gold white.**

Lucky Stones   **Ruby, amber, diamonds.**

Your Lucky Numbers 1, 10, 28, 37, 46, 55

HAPPINESS LIES IN POSITIVE LIVING
BE POSITVE THINK POSITIVE LIVE POSITIVE
CHAPTER SIX

ZODIAC SIGNS

VIRGO (23rd August to 22nd September)

Your Planetary Ruler   Mercury

Your Element   Earth

Your Sign   Movable

Characteristics

You are attractive, modest, reserved, honest, long armed, with drooping shoulders, sweet speech, intelligent, fond of pleasure, music and opposite sex.

Physical Appearance

Often of a small build, you have a large fund bustling energy and are seldom able to sit still for long. Your noses a seldom bulbous, and your lips are generally delicately shaped. Your sky tends to be soft and oily in your younger years.

Personality

You are discriminating, analytical, objective and practical. As a result, you excel in all work in which analysis and critical judgment is required. You have great clarity in your thoughts and strong powers of discerning hidden things. However, although you have a strong love for justice, you are only moderately sympathetic towards others. You are cool-headed and balanced. Happily, you are not vindictive and in fact, quite shy, prefer to work quietly and in seclusion. You are likely to travel a great deal for business or pleasure. Travel brings good luck and addition to fortune.

By and large, you will rise by dint of your personal efforts and merit. Once aroused, it's difficult for you to cool down. You also tend to live in your imagination far too often.

Profession and Career

You would do well in all occupations connected with higher sciences, mechanics, dietetics, nutrients, health, and labor. Since you go into details, you are industrious, and are devoted to your work. You make good executives, organizers and directors. You are an earthy sign, and if you have an inclination for agriculture and horticulture, you can successful in any occupation connected with land.

Business and Finances

Acquisition of wealth will prove an uphill task. Though the struggle will be hard and beset with many difficulties, you will triumph ultimately due to intelligent handling and hard work. You will, however, have secret enemies, and should be very careful in your investments.

Ideal Match

Taurus, Virgo and Capricorn.

Romance and Marriage

Your love life is not smooth as a rule, partly because you have high expectations always. There are, chances of second marriage. Even if there is no second marriage, there may be a long-standing attachment. Many of you have a tendency to fall in love at a comparatively young age, but such a relationship is seldom enduring.

Health and Disease

Your health is, generally, not good in childhood, but as the years pass, and it becomes better. You are likely to have complaints of the bowels and weakness of the sympathetic nervous system, the abdomen and the liver, the gall bladder and gall ducts. Virgos are very fussy food eaters. You are anemic and suffer from indigestion, gas pains, ulcers, liver upsets, and colitis and bowel problems

Lucky Days   **Wednesday, Saturday.**

Lucky Colors   **Orange, Yellow, Grey, White.**

Lucky Stones   **Emerald, Jade, amethyst, topaz.**

Your Lucky Numbers 5, 14, 50, 59 68 and 77

HAPPINESS LIES IN POSITIVE LIVING
BE POSITVE THINK POSITIVE LIVE POSITIVE
CHAPTER SEVEN

ZODIAC SIGNS

LIBRA (23rd September to 22nd October)

Your ruling planet   **Venus**

Your Element   **Air**

Your sign   **Movable**

CHARACTERISTIC

Libra being the seventh sign of the zodiac and is ruled by the Planet Venus. You are attractive, tall and have a very sharp nose. You are intelligent, learned, religious, lover of beautiful things of nature and fond of pleasures. AS you possess sound judgments you are clever at making schemes. You are quite popular, lover of Art and Music.

Physical Appearance

Physically, you don't appear to be too strong and robust at first glance but you actually have great stamina. Your skin usually has a healthy glow to it and people often envy the texture of your hair.

Personality

You are gentle, compassionate and have an affectionate nature. You are large-hearted, with strong passions. You have a keen sense of honor and justice. In case of a dispute, friends and acquaintances are likely to turn to you as an arbitrator.

If you are appointed as judges, you keep the scales even. You have a keen aesthetic sense as well, and are fond of beauty and symmetry. Your judgments are on the dot but sometimes, you tend to be hesitant and indecisive, preferring to err on the side of diplomacy and tact. You often achieve a good position in life due to unexpected assistance from relatives. In religious matters, you are broad-minded, and want to follow the good and moral tenets of all religions and philosophies. However, you meet serious opposition in life from people in the field of religion and law.

Profession

You succeed in law, art, music, dealing in merchandise, mechanics, or professions connected with wines, spirits and liquors, science and navigation. Advocates, you make good Actors, Judges, Politicians, Diplomats and Salespersons.

Business and Finances

You seldom find yourself in a position where you have to take a loan. You often come into riches through a marriage or by entering into a business partnership. You build up your finances step-by-step for the future, and purchase property by paying regular installments.

You Match with   Gemini, Libra or Aquarius.

Romance and Marriage

You are inclined to go through more than one relationship before deciding whom to marry. You are affectionate by nature, and make good friends. Sometimes your friendship is mistaken as love by the opposite sex. You should in fact avoid self-indulgence in matters of sex and affection, and should not enter into bonds of matrimony with the first person you like

Your weakness

You often spend your energy taking care of others instead of yourself. Plenty of water is necessary in a day for you as this keeps you away from toxins. Proper rest is very necessary for your health. So it would be advisable on your part to take proper rest and not to over exhort yourself.

Health and Disease

You are likely to suffer from diseases of the bowels, the bladder, the kidneys, the lumbar region, and the spine. At times, however, you tend to be a bit of a hypochondriac, worrying about your health and that of family members, even when no serious ailments are anywhere on the horizon. You are pretty healthy people but still you are prone to weakness in the lower back when you over exert yourself. You suffer from allergies, asthma and frequent colds and flu. The skin, hair, veins as well as throat, kidneys and lumbar region of you get easily affected.

Lucky Days   **Fridays, Mondays.**

Lucky Colors   **Blue, green and white.**

Lucky Stones   **Sapphire, Turquoise Opal.**

Your Lucky Numbers   **6, 15, 42, 51, 60**

HAPPINESS LIES IN POSITIVE LIVING
BE POSITVE THINK POSITIVE LIVE POSITIVE
CHAPTER EIGHT

ZODIAC SIGNS

SCORPIO   (24th October to 21st November)

Your Planetary Ruler   Mars Pluto

Your Element   Water

Your sign   Fixed

Characterizes

You have a well-set body and are of middle structure, you have a youthful appearance and are fickle minded fellow. You are clever powerful and dignified at the same time you are cruel, sensual and usually not generous. You are a good conversationalist and you possess equally good writing skills, and are of commanding nature.

Physical Appearance

Generally, you present an attractive and strikingly tidy appearance with not a hair out of place, your nails well cared for and so on. Most of you have a fine skin texture. However, once you have entered your thirties, you tend to put on weights.

Personality

You have a strong and dominating personality, with strong will power. Generally, you never forget a grudge, and take revenge even after a long time. You do not prefer a frontal attack, and opt for indirect means. Subtle strategies and conspiracies hold a special fascination for you.

Therefore, you must be specially beware of who may happen to be your enemies. You are not only subtle, but energetic too. Generally, people around you are quick to note that you have a keen and penetrating

Intellect, combined with great dynamism. You are also analytical, skillful and patient, and have literary abilities and creative talents.

Profession and Career

The most suitable professions for you are those related to music, art and scientific pursuits. You also do well as doctors, particularly, as surgeons in departments of public health. You make good Architects, Executives in Industry, Officers in the Military and Navy, Chemists, Heads of Institutions, Mechanical engineers, Machinists, Sales Managers.

Business and Finances

You are shrewd at business matters, and financially, you generally do well. But you like to make a lot of money all at once. You have to be patient and persevering in building your finances. You should adopt wait and watch policy rather than grabbing all the entire lot at one time.

Ideal Match   Cancer, Scorpio and Pisces.

Romance and Marriage

Love and Romance are the basic instincts of your harmful life. You are prone to get attraction of the opposite sex. In spite of your refusal to accept the pure love of the opposite sex you easily get on facial attraction rather than true love. You are considered very sexy and are intense lovers, with the attraction being more of physical craving than pure love. In several cases it has been noticed that probably there may be a tragedy in the first part of your life, and you may marry a second time.

Health and Disease

Your health calls for more care and attention. Since you are a good eater of delicious food you should be more careful in your choice of food. You are also prone to fevers and bruises. The weak parts in your anatomy are the groin and bladder, the pelvis, the stomach and the throat. You are prone to catching infections and contagious diseases.

Your Weakness

You generally put off things till the last moment and you also prepare at the eleventh hour it is because of your fortune that you come out successfully. You have the tendency to start late but again your fortune favors you to finish first. Though on the face it you appear to be frank playful and blunt but actually you would like to keep all secrets in your heart and mind.

Lucky Days   Tuesday and Thursday.

Lucky Colors   Rust, red, earth brown.

Lucky Stone

Bloodstone, Topaz, Garnet, Red Coral.

Your Lucky Numbers   9, 18, 36, 45,

HAPPINESS LIES IN POSITIVE LIVING
BE POSITVE THINK POSITIVE LIVE POSITIVE
CHAPTER NINE
ZODIAC SIGNS

SAGITTARIUS (22nd November to 21st December)

Your Planetary Ruler   **Jupiter**

Your Element   **Fire**

Your sign   **Movable**

Character tics

You are well known for your boldness and dashing approach in relationship and conversations. You are courageous pushy and accommodating. You being a dual sign you believe in that variety is this spice of life. You also insist on your personal freedom and liberty.

Appearance

Generally fine boned with a glowing complexion, large eyes, a pert nose and a charming smile, you tend to walk with a gliding movement. Your bodily actions are Usually soft and refined instead of being clumsy and ungainly.

Personality

You are usually quite brilliant, noble and refined. You are swift and sudden in speech and action. Sometimes you speak out your mind even before the other person has finished a sentence. You are truthful, and keep your promises. You are bold, free and dashing. You make friends easily, and are attached to them.

You are socially successful, and many persons of high standing will become your patrons. But some of them will prove to be highly treacherous, and will almost result in your loss of position. Your enemies will prove to be very bitter and persistent. You should take care that your position and prosperity are not threatened by the mischief of your enemies. You have a strong instinct, and are more successful if you work according to your own instincts, rather than on the advice of others. You should avoid betting, speculation and gambling, as this habit may lead to heavy losses.

Profession and Career

You can succeed well in teaching, in the field of religion and law, in politics, administration, and also in business or banking. You are good sports persons, fond of hunting and the outdoor life and would do well in any occupation connected with them. You have a strong dramatic sense as well, and can also do well in occupations connected with the stage.

Business and Finances

Your early years will not be prosperous. You may be subjected to financial stringency on account of losses your parents may have suffered. Success will come to you only after middle age. Up to your thirtieth year, you are likely to have frequent setbacks in your financial career. But success does come to you, as your sun sign is ruled by Jupiter, which stands for honor, riches and position. You do not have a strong inclination towards purchase of real estate and immovable properties. Consequently, very few persons born under this sun sign build large estates.

Ideal Match   Aries, Leo, Sagittarius and Pisces.

Romance and Marriage

In choosing your spouse, you are more idealistic than passionate. Consequently, even after the engagement, you break off the relationship if you find that your finance is not up to your mark. You love, but since you are not demonstrative in your affections, others may misunderstand them as lacking in warmth. However, if your spouse fails to keep in pace with you, the marriage may break. At times, there are two marriages, one of which proves detrimental to your progress.

Health and Disease

Your general health is good, but you are likely to suffer from nervous disorders. The sign Sagittarius rules the hips, thighs and the muscular system. It is also connected with the motor impulses. You are likely to suffer from mental tension, Sciatica, Hip Disease or some kind of lameness.

YOUR WEAKNESS

You being a masculine sing, you do not hesitate to think and you speak out and act, as you desire. Though you are truthful in your thoughts people will misunderstand and take you as their enemies because of your harsh and bold talks, you will speak out what you feel is right without considering how the others would value your such statements. You are advice not to be out spoken if you want to maintain your relationship with others.

Lucky Days	**Monday and Thursday**
Lucky Colors	**Red, Pink, and Purple.**
Lucky Stones	**Topaz, and Turquoise. Your**
Lucky Numbers	**3, 12, 21, 39, 48**

HAPPINESS LIES IN POSITIVE LIVING
BE POSITVE THINK POSITIVE LIVE POSITIVE
CHAPTER TEN

ZODIAC SIGNS

CAPRICORN (22nd December to 19thJanuary)

Your Planetary Ruler   Saturn

Your Element   Earth

Your sign   Moveable

Characteristics

You will be economical, prudent, reasonable, thoughtful and practical in life. You will be calculative and you will execute any work after taking a thoughtful and careful decision. You will have the required push and confidence and you will not hesitate in bringing through chance in your career, once you take a bold and careful decision you have a study nature, immense tolerance but at times you will lack the required degree of patience. You are serious in disposition, and humility is one of your chief characteristics.

Appearance

You are good looking, with sharp features, well shaped eyebrows and sensual lips. Your eyes are piecing in their intensity at times. You facial outlook is also quite pleasing and attraction.

Personality

You are prudent, cautious and hard working. You are active and vigorous, and, at the same time, plodding. You are endowed with a spirit of service, and have a strong sense of duty. You have initiative that brings you success. You are practical and economical in spending. You are loyal and conscientious in your work. Your practical nature, at times, gives the impression that you lack warmth. But actually, you are loving and devoted. You will meet opposition from persons occupying high or low ranks, but will, ultimately, surmount all obstacles. You will have powerful patronage of a very high personage, particularly, if you are in the armed forces. In service, you will give satisfaction to your superior. You often rise high in politics too.

Profession and Career

You succeed well in all occupations where hard work and plodding are the main features. You do well in work connected with Agriculture, Forestry, Education, Biology, in Factories and large organizations.

Business and Finances

You are versatile and shrewd in business. You earn money on your own and not due to any windfall, legacy or inheritance. Money also comes to you late in life. You have to toil pretty hard to get to the highest position in life. Money does not come to you that easily.

Ideal Match   Taurus, Virgo, Libra and Capricorn.

Romance and Marriage

You do not marry in a hurry, and do so only when you are assured that the other party reciprocates your love. However, you do not prove stable in your affections.

This is not due to an inborn unfaithful disposition but due to the influence of others. Your spouse may be fickle, and bring about a break in your marital relationship. Often, you prefer to marry a homebody who can provide home comforts and good companionship.

Health and Disease

You are likely to suffer from rheumatism or gout. You are liable to get liver trouble nervous tension should be avoided. Your stomach is weak spot. Your health gets better with your age. You tend to suffer from joint problems, arthritis, neuralgia and rheumatism. You are prone to skin diseases and have problems with bones, gall bladder, teeth and spleen.

Your Weakness

You often tend to become desperate, broken hearted and test yourself to a greater height where you feel the burden of physical strain. Therefore you should correct yourselves and you should be aware of others as well as your fault and deficiency you should avoid nervousness at all cost.

Lucky Days   **Saturday**

Lucky Colors   **Grey, black, blue, brown.**

Lucky Stones   **Blue Sapphire, Amethyst, Onyx.**

Lucky Numbers 1, 10, 4, 22, 35, 44

HAPPINESS LIES IN POSITIVE LIVING
BE POSITVE THINK POSITIVE LIVE POSITIVE
CHAPTER ELEVEN

ZODIAC SIGNS

AQUARIUS   **(20th January to 18th February)**

Your Ruling Planet   Saturn, Uranus

Your Element   Air

Born in Sign: Fixed

CHARACTERISTIC

Being the eleventh sign of the zodiac, you have a broad
outlook and human understanding. You are outspoken,
social, intelligent, and you possess good retentive
power. You are also shrewd, clever headed you have
your own way of thinking and doing things and you
carry out your works according to your own discretion.
You will not hesitate to do any unusual or irregular
thing even if you consider tobe morally upright. Your
sense of dressing and the taste of clothing would be
something different and you not like to imitate others.
You have your individuality, mannerism peculiarity and
your own specialty. You are often far ahead with fresh
ideas and schemes. You generate new ideas and at

times act in a way which shows that the laws are not made for you which means you over act and your actions are beyond anything body's imagination. You develop good intuition and mental will prefer to go for deep meditation and good concentration.

Appearance

You are middle stature strong person and have broad shoulder and large bones with a little amount of grace and your physical appearance is quite striking. Quite of you possess high cheeks and a peculiar winning smile.

Personality

You have an alert mind, and are keen to acquire more knowledge. You have striking intuitive and psychic powers. You possess a strong will power, and are hard working. You are fond of solitude, and are patient and persevering in your efforts. You are religious and philosophical. You see religion and philosophy as a manifestation of beauty and harmony, a means of universal love and service to mankind. You have a logical mind, and would do well to be guided by your own intuition and reasoning rather than that of others in arriving at decisions. You are kind hearted, original, simple, energetic and systematic. You are honest to your friends and enjoy enormous respect in your group. Your friends and contacts will range from many influential and eminent people yet you will feel melancholy and lonely at times. You will be ready to help others at the moment's notice but will always remain personally detached. You are an idealist independent, inventive thinker, quick witted, positive, and excitable and, when need be you are also aggressive and combative.

Profession and Career

Since you a scientific bent of mind the profession and career best suited for you are Finance Marketing, Administration, Writing, Physiologists, Acting and you excel well when you are given the chance to handle most difficult situation or posts. You are also excellent when it comes to public dealing and can speak well in public Meetings. You do well as Leaders, Managers and Bosses.

Business and Finances

You are not so keen on building your bank balance, yet you do save money, which you are inclined to use for the benefit of the public at large. You have a strong desire to possess a second house, such as a country home.

 You are fond of traveling, but one of these journeys will be the cause of financial reverses or loss in social position. You have very good relations with your servants and employees. But you should be careful that the latter do not cause you any financial harm.

You match with   Gemini, Libra or Aquarius.

Romance and Marriage

Your domestic life is usually gets disturbed when you tend to lose your mental balance. Your love affairs will have a strong intellectual and artistic bias. Since you are very idealistic, you will have to be adaptable in your matrimonial relationship, even if you find that your partner does not come up to your standard. Your spouse will have an artistic temperament but is likely to be proud and imperious.

Health and Disease

You suffer from high blood pressure, hardening of arteries and Circulatory problems. Your sign rules nervous and lymphatic systems the ankles, calves of the legs, and throat, lungs, heart. You have a strong constitution, but are liable to fall ill suddenly, and such illnesses affect your nervous system. Precautions should also be taken against infectious diseases. You have a tendency to put on weight if you are not careful. You are also prone to sinus and bladder infections, varicose veins and cramps in lower legs.

YOUR WEAKNESS

Since you are over sensitive, your feelings are easily hurt .You often tend to loose control of yourself and do undesirable acts or things which you regret later. Though you are quite social yet you suffer from loneliness at times. In personal life you often indulge in lovely romantic affairs or extra marital affairs, which make your married life unhappy.

Lucky Days   Sunday, Saturday

Lucky Colors

Purple, Grey, black, blue, bluish green.

Lucky Stone   Sapphire, aquamarine, opal, onyx.

Your Lucky Numbers   4, 13, 22, 31, 40, 49.

HAPPINESS LIES IN POSITIVE LIVING
BE POSITVE THINK POSITIVE LIVE POSITIVE
CHAPTER TWELVE
ZODIAC SIGNS

PISCES   (19th February to 20th March)

Your Planetary Ruler   Jupiter, Neptune

Your Element   Water

Your sign   Fixed

Characteristics

You will be philosophical, restless, contemplating, imagining, honest, outspoken and helpful. You will be sweet tempered and socially inclined towards others. You being a common and famine sign your expression and thoughts will be modified and even thoroughly changed when you are in front of the audience you will have the desire to study the occult science and the divine life of god.

Appearance

You are generally of short stature with a tendency to be plump, short limbs, a full face, pale complexion, a tendency to develop a double chin, muscular and spherical shoulders. You have big and protruding eyes, soft and silky hair and a wide mouth.

Personality

You have a kind, loving, truthful and sympathetic nature. Usually, you are courteous and hospitable, helpful and humane, and you cannot harm any one even if you try. Being a dual sign, you are a puzzle to others and even to yourself. By and large, you are sweet tempered and social.

Professions and Career

You can be successful as accountants, bankers, as performers in music and opera houses, cinema, practitioners of occult sciences, actors, liaison officers, personnel in medical and education departments.

Business and Finances

You have good business ability. You are end owed with skills, which will bring you wealth and power. You do not relish the idea of being dependent on your children in old age so you keep the money safe for that period. You are helpful to needy people but mostly make advances of money to those who can repay on demand. You have plurality of interests.

Romance and Marriage

You are strongly attracted to romance and look for a combination of good looks and intellect in your partner. However, you tend to be suspicious by nature towards your partner, which can kill your love. You are easily taken in by flattery, and should not select a partner who sets too much store on socialization.

Ideal Match   **Virgo, Cancer and Pisces.**

Health and Diseases

Your mostly inclined to suffer from Nervous, Depression, Insomnia Anemia and Eye trouble.

Your Weakness

You are have the quality to speak and understand the domestic difficulties of the poor and will go about to assist them in the need of their hour but without considering your own financial position. The main weakness in you that you will rely upon all your friends and you will realize late in your life that your friends have not withstood to your expectation.

You are advised not to keep contemplating and daydreaming.

Lucky Days   **Monday, Tuesday and Thursday**

Lucky Colors   **Yellow, and Orange**

Lucky Stones   Yellow Sapphire, Opal and Ruby

Lucky Numbers 2, 11, 22, 31, 40

HAPPINESS LIES IN POSITIVE LIVING

BE POSITVE THINK POSITIVE LIVE POSITIVE

CHAPTER THIRTEEN

HOW TO CREATE POSITIVITY THROUGH

COMPATABILITY OF ZODIAC SIGNS

ZODIAC SIGNS

ARIES   WITH OTHER ZODIAC   SIGNS

ARIES WITH ARIES

An Aries female tends to dominate and if one person will submit to the other there should be much compatibility between two persons born in this fire sign. If both Arians have dominant and forceful aspects in their horoscopes, conflict will arise, as both partners desire to be head of the family. The situation dictates that both shall go for their own careers or directions independently. What starts out so promisingly ends in disharmony? A divorce can be rather be violent and heart breaking.

There in order to lead a happy and peaceful life they both have to submit to each other their likes and dislikes.

ARIES WITH TAURUS

Aries is impulsive, but Taurus is steady. Both are highly sensual, but the deliberate teasing and unpredictable lovemaking of Taurus can annoy Aries. Taurus is possessive and views Aries's need to be an individual desire rather than individual demand. Taurus is good at earning money but Aries is more spend thrift. This match may not make a fine combination as Venus, the goddess of love, rules Taurus nature and Mars the fiery planet rules Aries. Taurus being slow moving may find the going a bit hectic, though excitement may help to stimulate the friendship but this friendship may not be a lasting affair. Arians tend to omit their temperamental outbursts. Taurus is not highly emotional on the surface, but they can become furious as a bull, as and when they see red in Aries.

ARIES WITH GEMINI

They won't bore each other because as both love to talk more. Gemini is versatile and ingenious and Aries is dynamic and intelligent. They share a special compatibility, for Gemini is as restless and anxious to try new things as Aries is. Gemini is clever enough to counter Aries's needs. The signals are definitely go. Aries is likely to be the leader sexually, and Gemini delights in thinking up variations to keep Aries's interest at a peak. Gemini being a mercurial sign, where the mind plays an important part in all love making, and the emotional Arian may be too much for the conventional nature of the Gemini. This combination sometimes has a great deal of hankering because of strong differences in their personalities. It is not a great match up.

ARIES WITH CANCER

These two are fascinated with each other. Cancer is cautious. Cancer loves heart and home and Aries hates to be tied down. Resentments often build up and they argue over petty mattes. Aries has a sharp tongue that wounds the Cancerians. This combination is usually hard to match. The moon rules Cancerians, making them moody, sentimental and secretive. Their tendency is to live in the past, and they have a difficult time forgetting serious quarrels or disagreement that may occur occasionally this is quite true of this couple.

ARIES WITH LEO

This is usually a great combination. But both have got egos problems and both like to lead. Aries wouldn't dream of taking second place, and Leo needs constant watch. They can work it out properly if neither tries to defame the other. Though it's a fine sexual match, as both are fiery and romantic. Aries is optimistic and open to life; Leo is generous and good-hearted. They could find room to compromise easily as with both sides being emotional in their make up, Leo will fascinate an Arian mate if Aries will allow Leo to hold the centre of the floor on occasions. Their sex life could be legendary and infidelity kept to a minimum, or eliminated altogether if each of them find what they want from each other, and not have a physical compulsion to stray. Leo admires the aggressive tendencies of fiery signs. That is why Arians make this an ideal union.

ARIES WITH VIRGO

Mercury rules Virgo and Aries is ruled by Mars. But they have totally different ideas. Aries's passions are impulsive and direct. Virgo's sexuality is more enigmatic and takes time to be revealed. In other areas Aries is full of exciting new plans and ideas, and insists on being boss. Virgo is critical and fussy, and likes things to be done the way he wants. They end up making war, not love and do not blend well astrologically. Virgos desire a well-ordered existence and won't be happy under Arian leadership. If the Arian allows Virgo space, and acknowledges the virtues of Virgo, the two can make for a dynamic relationship.

ARIES WITH LIBRA

Libra wants peace, quiet, and harmony while Aries wants action and adventure. Both like social life, entertaining, and pleasure, but both are restless in their ways. There is a powerful initial attraction between these two but their love life may be bit unconventional. Libra will look for someone less demanding, and Aries will bind someone for more dictating.

Marvelous affair but poor marriage shows. Libra's refined and artistic temperament wishes for reciprocal attachments. And this is something Aries cannot provide. There is a wider the ordinary margin for error though, and most of these combinations will go at the distance and nonreciprocal.

ARIES WITH SCORPIO

With Mars dominating both signs it makes for very positive temperaments unless there are some bad natal planetary aspects. Since Aries won't take orders from Scorpions and Scorpio will never take a back seat. Love cannot be a bonfire between these two. Though they've physical, energetic, and passionate in their sexual nature and each has a forceful personality and wants to control the other there is no room for these two. This combination is can make an ideal match if one ignores to dominate the other.

ARIES WITH SAGITTARIUS

The Mars-Jupiter duo is usually an ideal match for each other. Sagittarius is a perfect ideal and temperamental match for Aries. They both are active, spontaneous people. There may be a little conflict because both are impulsive and brutally frank. However, they have wonderful senses of humor and enjoy each other's company. If they make it in the bedroom, they'll make it everywhere else. Most people of these matches are in it for life. The Sagittarius means liberty, and the pursuit of happiness while Aries is subscribes to this theory. And for this reason, that makes them a good match

ARIES WITH CAPRICORN

Capricorns are usually patient and are traditionally easygoing. Arians are too impatient to cope with the slowness attitude. Saturn represents the Capricorn and Mars governs the Aries. Aries's taste for innovation and experiment may not please Capricorns. Aries is restless, fiery, and impulsive; Capricorn is ordered, settled, and practical. Capricorn needs to dominate and so does Aries. Problems often crops up over moneymaking schemes. Not a hopeful combination. Capricorn will nod against the Arian will and a disagreement is bound to occur. In the matter of sex there is an affinity; however, their inherent personalities clash. The combination of a fire sign with an earth sign. Aries is a fiery in nature while Capricorn is earth, cautious and reserved. Aries prefers to take action while Capricorn would rather plan and wait. Without a great deal of tolerance and patience, there is not much hope for this union

ARIES WITH AQUARIUS

Both signs are of independent nature but at times Aquarius will do things without notice with which Aries may become impatient. Since both are active, ambitious, enjoy a wide range of interests, and are equally eager for sexual adventure. As both are independent Aquarius energies more than Aries and Aries may at times feel neglected. Aries finds the Aquarian unpredictability exciting, but feels entirely insecure. However, with a bit of tact and understanding on both sides, this is a great affair that could turn into something even better. This could possibly be a good relationship, but will require a positive attitude on both parts.

ARIES WITH PISCES

Pisceans are romantic and they desire the delicate approach that which the Arian lacks. Aries will draw Pisces out of their shell, and in turn will be appealed by Pisces mysterious nature in terms of sexuality. The boldness and confidence of Aries adding to the Pisces's intuitions and fantasies end in an eventful union. Pisces is somewhat shy and Aries likes to be dominant, Pisces likes having someone to be looked upon. For a happy coupling thus requires only a little more tact on Ariean part.

HAPPINESS LIES IN POSITIVE LIVING

BE POSITVE THINK POSITIVE LIVE POSITIVE

CHAPTER FOURTEEN

HOW TO CREATE POSITIVITY THROUGH

COMPATABILITY OF ZODIAC SIGNS

ZODIAC SIGNS

TAURUS WITH ARIES

Taurus is possessive and views Aries's need to be an individual desire rather than individual demand. Aries is an impatient, energetic sign, rather domineering the slower-moving Taurus may find the going a bit hectic, but the excitement may help stimulate courtship since Taurus is a highly emotional sign, though very obstinate when dictated to. Taurean nature is ruled by Venus, the goddess of love, and Aries is ruled by Mars the fiery planet. Aries is impulsive, but Taurus is steady. Both are highly sensual, but the deliberate teasing and unpredictable lovemaking of Taurus can annoy Aries. This match may not make a fine combination as Taurus being slow moving may find the going a bit hectic, though excitement may help to stimulate the friendship but this friendship may not be a lasting affair.

TAURUS WITH TAURUS

Both are earthy creatures that prefer safety to adventure. From a physical stand point; this appears to be a compatible combination. Both share a fondness for money, and are hardworking, loyal, and affectionate.

The female Taurean tends to be more sentimental than the male Taurean, but each is as possessive than the other, which works out fine. Because they are both earthy and direct about sexual needs, there should be no problem in that department, if one adheres to the will and wishes of the other.

TAURUS WITH GEMINI

The Gemini personality may prove to be too restless for the Taurus nature. The two signs are emotionally at distance. These two are completely unalike in temperament. Taurus is fixed in opinions, resistant to change. Gemini is restless, vacillating. Gemini is attracted to Taurus's passions, but in time Taurus's instinct for security and stability will be offended by Gemini volatile nature. Taurus's demands are simply too much for Gemini, who seeks excuses. Taurus with the innate need to possess will never be able to hang on to the unsettled Gemini. Gemini loves change and Taurus resists it so becomes rather difficult for both of them to come to an understanding in the matters of making love.

TAURUS WITH CANCER

Usually this makes a good combination. Cancer likes a good home with much affection. This is what every Taurean hopes to find when undertaking conventional responsibilities. Cancer needs someone like Taurus to depend on as Cancer gives Taurus the loyalty and feedback it needs. Taurus is ambitious for money and security, and Cancer has exactly those same goals. Similar interests and desires make for harmonious meetings. From an emotional point of view, there is nothing in the stars that bars the prospect of a happy married life between these two partners. This is a good combination as both signs are naturally attracted by the others sense for feelings and emotions.

TAURUS WITH LEO

Venus and the Sun make a good combination, especially when each understands the other's faults. Excellent physical qualities and great attraction is there for both partners. Taurus will supply the attention that Leo requires but will expect it to be returned. A strong attraction physically and emotionally but having too many obstacles to cope with.

TAURUS WITH VIRGO

With both being earth signs there will be much common ground for these two. Both Virgo and Taurus desire material success and security. Taurus keeps a careful eye on expenditures, which pleases Virgo. Although they lack what might be called a spontaneous approach to life, neither puts a high value on that. Both share the same intellectual pursuits. Taurus's attraction and Virgo's sharp mind are a good combination for success as a team.

TAURUS WITH LIBRA

Libra an air sign loves to roam and Taurus an earth sign loves to sit and waits patiently. With understanding it could be a harmonic relationship. Taurus balances Libra's indecisiveness. Taurus finds Libra a warm, romantic, partner. Libra is born to charm. The love goddess and it does shine on the two lovebirds that are until one-steps out of line. Both signs are ruled by Venus and have sensual natures, but each expresses this quality differently. However there are common interest and a meeting of the mind and body making this a very good marital combination. They appreciate beauty and the finer things of life.

TAURUS WITH SCORPIO

These two are opposites in the zodiac, but they have more in common than other opposites. Both are determined and ambitious, and neither is much of a lover. These are zodiac opposites, but they are compatible earth and water signs. This usually manifests itself in a strong physical attraction. This combination mutually admires each other. Jealousy however is the big problem with this pair and that seems to be always showing its face. Taurus must be careful to keep faith with the scorpion, or else this combination will fall down without warning.

TAURUS WITH SAGITTARIUS

These are two very different personality types the more reserved Taurus and the outgoing Sagittarius both has an appreciation for the truth. Sagittarius has an easy live and let live attitude this might work if Taurus can tie a string to Sagittarius's.

The Taurus who marries a Sagittarian will find that no amount of arguing or berating is going to change the reckless Sagittarian With some understanding they can find harmony in their characters as long as they allow each other their personalities. With the Taurean being possessive and the Sagittarian being freedom loving, the Sagittarian may find this hard to co-operate with.

TAURUS WITH CAPRICORN

A good combination of the basic earth signs. Both are responsible and practical natures. They even have a mutual desire for success and material things. Capricorn is a strong match for Taurus, for they both have passions that are straightforward and uncomplicated. Capricorn is a bit more secretive than Taurus. With both partners having mutual understanding of each other's personalities this can be a very compatible marriage. Venus and Saturn blend very well from an emotional point of view.

TAURUS WITH AQUARIUS

These two live on opposite sides of the planet, in fact some times, Taurus will wonder if Aquarius is even from this planet. Neither is likely to approve of the other. Taurus is conservative, careful, closemouthed. Aquarius is unconventional, innovative, and vivacious. Taurus is lusty and passionate while Taurus needs security and comfort. Aquarius, a fancy-free loner who resents ties that bind. This combination heads in for many difficulties. The Aquarian being unpredictable both love ease and comfort but their views on how to obtain them are very different. Another big irritation for the Taurus lover is the unwillingness of the Aquarius to share his secrets. Aquarius will find the Taurus attention somewhat smothering and restrictive.

TAURUS WITH PISCES

These two can share a great deal of their appreciation for beauty, art, and sensuality and just about any of the finer things in life. Pisces may not altogether understand Taurus's materialistic approach to life. Taurus's practical, easygoing nature helps Pisces through its frequent changes of mood.

In love, Taurus is devoted and Pisces adores. This usually is a very happy combination. Pisces being romantic, imaginative, impressionable and flexible is just what the Taurus native is looking for.

HAPPINESS LIES IN POSITIVE LIVING
BE POSITVE THINK POSITIVE LIVE POSITIVE

CHAPTER FIFTEEN

HOW TO CREATE POSITIVITY THROUGH

COMPATABILITY OF ZODIAC SIGNS

ZODIAC SIGNS

GEMINI WITH ARIES

Gemini respects the refined, intellectual approach to continual bliss. Impatient Arians may find this frustrating, after a while may try to find a less difficult companion. This lively, energetic pair can be good friends as well as good lovers. Aries will probably make the decisions because Gemini has difficulty in that area. Not a great match up, but can work with understanding and effort. Aries needs to calm down. Don't get me wrong. Gemini is versatile and ingenious and Aries is dynamic and intelligent. They share a special compatibility, for Gemini is as restless and anxious to try new things as Aries is. Gemini is clever enough to counter Aries's needs. Gemini being a mercurial sign, where the mind plays an important part in all love making, and the emotional Arian may be too much for the conventional nature of the Gemini. It is not a great match up.

GEMINI WITH TAURUS

The Gemini personality may prove to be restless for the Taurean nature. Taurus wants life to be stables and ordered, while Gemini is easily bored and looks for new experiences. These two are completely unalike in temperament. Taurus's demands are simply and Gemini seeks excuses. Gemini loves change and Taurus resists it so becomes rather difficult for both of them to come to an understanding in the matters of understanding each other. An unpromising match.

GEMINI WITH GEMINI

As both are of air signs and are ruled by the planet mercury. These two will never bore each other, for they are interested in everything. A compatible combination this should prove to be, at least both would understand each other's changeable nature. The Gemini demands for change and variety will keep this relationship some how moving. Whether it produces a happiness or sadness depends on at least one of the companion paying attention, at least for some time. Discussions will be lively and ever changing life may become restless but again they cannot have it in any other way.

GEMINI WITH CANCER

Cancer needs security and homely atmosphere whereas Gemini dislikes to be being tied down. These two have too little in common for a long-term relationship. Gemini lacks patience with Cancer's moods and Gemini's sharp tongue is too harsh for Cancer's strong ego. While Gemini is constantly on the alert for change, Cancer is satisfied to become a truly homely mate. Cancers are driven by emotion and feelings and generally prefer to be constant. Gemini's unstoppable movement may prove be unsettling to Cancer's needs. They are poised for a downward trend. Gemini makes Cancer feel quite insecure and their affair is likely to result in a volatile behaviour.

GEMINI WITH LEO

On the surface there is great mutual attraction for both signs. While Leo loves with his heart first, Gemini loves with his mind.

Both are naturally attracted to glamour and flattery of the world. Their affair is a chase after variety and amusement. An affectionate pair who really enjoy each other. Leo will probably demand more adoration than Gemini is willing to give. Socially, each tries to upstage the other, but they have a lot of fun together doing it. There is good reason to be optimistic about this pairing; all in all this is a very good combination of air and fire.

GEMINI WITH VIRGO

Both are Mercury-ruled and have a mental approach to life. They are attracted to each other because of a mutual interest in intellectual ideas. Both have active minds. Virgo's analytical approach seems like indifference to Gemini. Virgo looks on Gemini's busy social life as superficial and a waste of time. Virgo is critical; Gemini is tactless. Mercury is calculating and logical; in Virgo it is critical and demanding. Gemini's ever-present desire for change would be much for the realistic Virgo. One point for the two to be compatible would be the desire for good clothes, cleanliness, mutual desire for friends and associates who are engaged in intellectual and artistic pursuits. Gemini can deal with Virgo's critical eye, well, this could work.

GEMINI WITH LIBRA

These two air signs are well suited in every way. Both signs have much in common and enough to make an ideal partnership. Libra being under Venus's influence and Mercury ruling Gemini makes for a very good planetary combination. This will be a very stimulating relationship. One sign compliments the other and brings out the better part of each other's nature. Gemini will find it easy to communicate with Libra who is only too happy to share his information and ideas. They are affectionate, fun loving, entertaining, and travel fond. This is considered to be a great astrological influence for a long and happy marriage.

GEMINI WITH SCORPIO

An air sign with a water sign. Gemini is too changeable and inconstant for intense Scorpio, who needs and demands total commitment. Scorpio is basically a loner; Gemini likes to glitter in social settings.

Gemini has a strong penchant for independence, while Scorpio wants to dominate and possess. Gemini's desire for freedom of action will clash with the jealous and possessive nature of Scorpio. While some Gemini-Scorpio combinations may work out fairly well, the pure Gemini- Scorpio alliance packs as much power as an atomic bomb. These two will have some difficulty rectifying their innate natures. Love conquers all. Then again, too much, stifles some. These two are opposites in the zodiac and are attracted to each other like magnets. They'll especially enjoy each other's minds for both have wide-ranging and varied interests.

GEMINI WITH SAGITTARIUS

Gemini is ruled by Mercury and Sagittarius is ruled by Jupiter the planet of knowledge and wisdom. Both have bright minds, but Sagittarius is outspoken while Gemini likes to enjoy fun. They are usually a compatible combination with both being frank, outspoken, and a certain amount of personal understanding being made. They meet on a common ground, and can plan their lives with equilibrium. They are restless, adventuresome, imaginative, and fun loving. No other opposite signs in the zodiac enjoy each other more than these two. However if Sagittarius forgoes its ego and Gemini restores to concrete planning they can make a good combination otherwise their combination may not last long.

GEMINI WITH CAPRICORN

Capricorn gets worried about security, while Gemini feels about losing its liberty. The Saturn ruled Capricorn will be at differences with the Mercury ruled Gemini. Patience is a virtue with Capricorn, but it is not so with Gemini. Gemini's need for a survival does nothing to make Capricorn feel secure. Gemini's free talks, meets opposition from conservative Capricorn. Capricorn's great drive to execute will prove to be too much for the Gemini. Until they both are ready to minimize their goals. Capricorn will go on hunting until he gains the upper hand. Of course with these two people going together anything is possible and the outcome of the result may not be satisfying to each other.

GEMINI WITH AQUARIUS

Gemini is bit inconstant or unstable, Aquarius understands somewhat Gemini's needs. Gemini is always looking for surprises and the Aquarian can give them. Gemini and Aquarius get along quite easily. They share a taste for new things, travelling, meeting new people and doing new things. Since both are unpredictable, things may always go smoothly with them. But love keeps getting them together, for Aquarius adores Gemini's wit and good cheer. The caring, thoughts of Aquarius will find a smooth home with Gemini. Uranus, the ruling planet of Aquarius, is full of surprises and sudden changes. This will suit the Gemini perfectly. There will be plenty of none stop variety to afford the stimulation that Gemini needs for its dual personality and goal.

GEMINI WITH PISCES

Their passion is quite high, and so are their problems. Pisces get easily hurt by thoughtless Gemini. Gemini is mischievous and playful, but Pisces is sensitive and takes things to heart easily. Each practices in his or her thoughts in their own way: Gemini needs freedom and Pisces needs unending appreciation. Pisces just can't feel secure with talkative moods of Gemini, and he tries to pull the net in his own way. This atmosphere eventually makes it hard for Gemini to breathe his own liberty. The freedom of Gemini is stake if he marries a Piscean. Gemini's should be prepared to change their ways if they want to seek happiness with a loving and possessive Piscean.

HAPPINESS LIES IN POSITIVE LIVING
BE POSITVE THINK POSITIVE LIVE POSITIVE

CHAPTER SIXTEEN

HOW TO CREATE POSITIVITY THROUGH

COMPATABILITY OF ZODIAC SIGNS

ZODIAC SIGNS

CANCER WITH ARIES

The moon rules Cancer, making him moody, sentimental and secretive. Aries is ruled by mars and makes him bold and aggressive. Cancer is easily hurt by Aries's aggressiveness and sharp tongue. Cancer likes security and Aries needs freedom to explore new worlds. Both like to accumulate money. Aries wants to spend it and Cancer wants to keep it. Too many problems here. This combination is usually hard to match. Cancer holds on like that of a crab, while Aries cannot part with the things so easily that are with them. The secretive nature of Cancer has the potential of clashing with the openness of Aries. Though Aries can be moody too, it is not quite so bad as Cancer. If they make it through the first year or so the rest may turn out to be an easy affair.

CANCER AND TAURUS

This is a good combination as both signs are naturally attracted to each other. Both need security and both are loving, affectionate, and passionate. Both are moneymakers, and together they enjoy the delights of heart and home. Taurus is good for Cancer's moodiness. What each needs the other supplies?

From an emotional point of view, there is nothing in the stars that bars the prospect of a happy married life between these two partners. One thing is what Tureen should remember is that Cancer is sensitive, and will crawl into a shell if he or she is unhappy emotionally.

CANCER AND GEMINI

Gemini is constantly on the alert for change, Cancer is satisfied to become a true mate. Cancer's nature is emotional and Gemini's nature is openness and that makes it difficult for them to understand each other. Cancer will try to keep Gemini penned in, and Gemini can't abide that. Cancer and moodiness may become too much for Gemini to cope with. There would be better compatibility where the female is a Gemini and the male is a Cancerian, Cancers are driven by emotion and feelings and generally prefer to remain constant while Gemini's unstoppable movement and talkative nature will prove unpleasant to Cancer desire.

CANCER AND CANCER

They understand each other perfectly and can also wound each other without even trying hard or harsh. Both are too sensitive, demanding and dependent. They have a lot in common, and each needs an enormous amount of attention. That's the main drawback and trouble. This combination can make married life easy going, because each will have a sympathetic understanding for the other's moods, and wishes. Though there are times were they may disagree, with each clinging to their previous experience and teachings each will no doubt understand the other better. Both will give enough consideration to their company and they should have no trouble in finding constant happiness.

CANCER AND LEO

Usually this is a good combination, since the Cancer reflects the light of the Leo. Leo's heart will soon forgive the mood outbursts that Cancer shows from time to time. Leo will appreciate cancer's attention and as long as cancer can forgive and forget that they feel neglected at times. Cancer will feel a bit more enthused around Leo and will probably let Leo run things.

Cancer has to get used to Leo's generous, open heartedness. Leo is just what insecure Cancer is looking for. Cancer's marvelous intuitions tell it exactly how to handle this Leo.

CANCER AND VIRGO

Virgo's demands may be a bit much for Cancer's desire for peace and quiet. Cancer's response is emotive while Virgo's is analytical. Cancer may have to warm up Virgo a little, since there is fire under the ice. This can turn into a comfortable and affectionate relationship. Cancer's struggle for financial security works perfectly with Virgo. Cancer's dependency neatly complements Virgo's need to protect, and each is anxious to please the other. The full, affectionate feelings of cancer will not be completely satisfied by Virgo's direct approach to the practical matters at hand. Virgo will appreciate the loyalty and sincerity of cancer, but will need to be a little more demonstrative and affectionate with cancer.

CANCER AND LIBRA

Cancer is not temperamentally suited to cope with the freedom loving Libran. This pair operates on entirely different levels. Cancer is too temperamental and possessive for airy Libra. They both love a beautiful home, but Libra also needs parties and people and outside pleasures. When Cancer turns critical, especially about Libra's extravagance, Libra starts looking elsewhere. On the positive side though, they could make it. Ruled by the Moon and Venus respectively, there is common ground here despite the fact that we have a water sign and an air. Libra will appreciate Cancer's loyalty and generosity. Cancer wants love Libra seeks perfect intellectual communion.

CANCER AND SCORPIO

Water signs rule both. Cancer is loyal; Scorpio's jealousy isn't provoked. Cancer admires Scorpio's strength while Scorpio finds a haven in Cancer's emotional commitment. Both are extremely intuitive and sense what will please the other. Together they can build a happy home where they feel safe and loved. This relationship has great intimacy, intensity, and depth. Things just get better all the time. Scorpio should make a good mate for quiet spoken cancer. Scorpio and cancer could well prove the ideal marriage combination.

CANCER AND SAGITTARIUS

A water and fire combination. Sagittarius likes to wander, while Cancer is a prefers to stay at home. Cancer's commitment to total togetherness only makes Sagittarius desperate to get away. In addition, outspoken Sagittarius's bluntness continually wounds sensitive Cancer. They happen to be better friends than lovers. There is a vast difference in natures and the likely hood of being compatible is all but impossible, unless there are some positive aspects in their charts. Cancer is too needy for Sagittarius. On the good side, they are both generous people.

CANCER AND CAPRICORN

Both signs have plenty in common. Capricorn has too many other interests to give Cancer all the attention it needs. Cancer is shy, sensitive, and needs affection, while Capricorn is aloof, and domineering. Capricorn has the ability to make cancer's dream come true, while Cancer is happy wishing for and wanting the success and security that the Capricorn strives for. The elements of water and earth go well together but these are zodiac opposites you can expect both side of the coin. They will have to take the good with the bad and there will be plenty of both. Capricorn lacks the warmth and sentiment that Cancer requires.

CANCER AND AQUARIUS

Cancer has a conservative taste while Aquarius taste is usually the opposite. Aquarius is quick-minded, unpredictable, and apt to be impatient with cautious, hesitant Cancer. Cancer needs to feel close and secure. The social side of the Aquarian may prove to be too much for the Cancer. Aquarian's love to share their life stories with the world while cancer is satisfied to concentrate on personal obligations. Odds against this combination are too great for this combination, unless one will become convergent to the other. Aquarius has a need to be independent and often appears detached in a close relationship with cancer.

CANCER AND PISCES

A harmonious match and quite a perfect match as both are ruled by the water signs.

The sentimental combination of these two signs make for an ideal marriage. Although both will have their moments of gloom and doom, they will soon come out in the sunshine to forgive and forget each other. They are both romantic, need to love and be loved and can probably communicate to each other without speaking or making facial gestures. Both are emotional, intensely devoted, and sensitive to each other's moods.

HAPPINESS LIES IN POSITIVE LIVING

BE POSITVE THINK POSITIVE LIVE POSITIVE

CHAPTER SEVENTEEN

HOW TO CREATE POSITIVITY THROUGH

COMPATABILITY OF ZODIAC SIGNS

LEO WITH OTHER ZODIAC SIGNS

LEO WITH ARIES

This is usually a great combination. But both have got egos problems and both like to lead. Aries wouldn't dream of taking second place, and Leo needs constant watch. They can work it out properly if neither tries to defame the other. Though it's a fine sexual match, as both are fiery and romantic. Aries is optimistic and open to life; Leo is generous and good-hearted. Leo admires the aggressive tendencies of fiery signs. That is why Arians make this an ideal union.

LEO WITH TAURUS

Leo requires but will expect it to be returned. Leo loves to dominate and eventually Taurus being strong willed but more patient.

Venus and the Sun make a good combination, especially when each understands the other's faults.

Excellent physical qualities and great attraction is there for both partners. Taurus will supply the attention that Leo requires but will expect it to be returned. A strong attraction physically and emotionally but having too many obstacles to cope with.

LEO WITH GEMINI

On the surface there is great mutual attraction for both signs. While Leo loves with his heart first, Gemini loves with his mind. Both are naturally attracted to glamour and flattery of the world. Their affair is a chase after variety and amusement. An affectionate pair who really enjoy each other. Leo will probably demand more adoration than Gemini is willing to give. Socially, each tries to upstage the other, but they have a lot of fun together doing it. There is good reason to be optimistic about this pairing; all in all this is a very good combination of air and fire. All in all this is a very good combination of air and fire.

LEO WITH CANCER

This is a combination of fire and water. Usually this is a good combination, since the Cancer reflects the light of the Leo. Leo's heart will soon forgive the mood outbursts that Cancer shows from time to time. Leo will appreciate cancer's attention and as long as cancer can forgive and forget that they feel neglected at times.

Cancer will feel a bit more enthused around Leo and will probably let Leo run things. Cancer has to get used to Leo's generous, open heartedness. Leo is just what insecure Cancer is looking for. Cancer's marvelous intuitions tell it exactly how to handle this Leo.

LEO WITH LEO

The both being fire signs. Two positive and strong willed individuals. Both are romantic, colorful, and exuberant about life. Each not only wants to sit on the throne, each wants to be the power behind it as well. They want to be the head of their social groups. The two are constantly competing for leadership; unhappy results can result from this. The only hope for a successful partnership is for the female to be content to rule the home and the male to shine in the business and social world.

It's difficult for one Leo to make room for another ego as large as its own, but that's exactly what's needed here.

LEO WITH VIRGO

Leo being a fire sign and Virgo being the earth sign. Here is a good chance for a happy partnership. Virgo is practical Leo is extravagant and a spendthrift. Leo likes to live life in a really big way, but Virgo is conservative. This is one of those relationships that depend on the type of relationship it is. Leo will overwhelm Virgo, whose criticism will irk Leo. In business it is best when Leo leads and Virgo follows and the differences will be tolerated. Both of them should look elsewhere. If Virgo will permit Leo to hold the limelight and refrain from being too critical they should have no real barriers to a happy and successful partnership. But this may be quite hard.

LEO WITH LIBRA

Leo being a fire and Libra being an air sign. The comparability of this two shall be tiring affair. The hale and hearty Leo may prove to be too much for the sensitive Libra nature, though they have a lot in common that could make for a good combination. The sun ruling Leo and Venus ruling Libra usually form a strong and luxurious aspect. Libra is indecisive and Leo will naturally take charge. Both signs love luxuries, are subject to flattery, and are very artistically inclined. The book may not always balance because they're both extravagant and love a beautiful setting in which to shine. Each will also try to outdo the other in order to get attention.

LEO WITH SCORPIO

Leo being a fire sign and Scorpio being water sign. Two very strong willed individuals generally create some rather stormy moments. But Leo finds it hard to cope with Scorpio's jealousy and possessiveness. Scorpio considers Leo a showpiece. Scorpio doesn't understand Leo's need to be continually surrounded by an admiring audience. Scorpio would rather dominate than admire, and that doesn't suit Leo's kingly state. Two shinning personalities join together. Basically this should make for one of the most compatible combinations, but long and happy partnership will be far better a Leo female marries a Scorpio male.

LEO WITH SAGITTARIUS

Both being of fire sign. The pendulum can swing in any body's favour. Together they share a liking for freedom, adventure, and meeting new people. Leo's natural quality of leadership brings out what loyalty Sagittarius can give. Leo is very proud, but self-confident and expansive Sagittarius is quite happy to let Leo go. Both love change and excitement and have a great zest for life.

LEO WITH CAPRICORN

Leo being a fire sign whereas Capricorn is an earth sign. The combination of these two may at time lead to severe complications. The slow Capricorn may prove to be too much for the carefree nature of Leo. Leo will think Capricorn stingy with affection because Capricorn's reserved, undemonstrative nature cannot give Leo the adoration it needs. Neither will take a back seat nor let the other dominate. This affair will be on the rocks before it even leaves the dock. Leo forgives and forgets; Capricorn being the one who is slow to anger and seldom forgets. This pair would not form the ideal basis for mutual understanding. Leo likes to live for the moment and Capricorn prefers to make calculated movements

LEO WITH AQUARIUS

Leo is a fire sign and Aquarius is an air sign. The comparability of this two in terms of worldly affairs can often become difficult to match. Both like socializing and meeting new people, but Leo always needs to perform on centre stage, which makes Aquarius impatient and irritable. Aquarius is too independent to become Leo's devoted subject. And that's where it ends. Leo views Aquarius's aloof emotions as a personal rejection. Both signs are better when doing things for others. Leo loves the world and Aquarius loves humanity. This makes for an excellent combination for a partnership that deals with or caters to the public. Each has a mutual understanding of the other when it comes to intimate matters, needs and desires.

LEO WITH PISCES

A Fire and water combination. Leo being a fire sign and Pisces being a water sign often makes this a unique combination.   Both are more inclined to take than to give. Fiery Leo and watery Pisces. This is the depiction of these two. Generally not expected to work but both have an ability to learn from one another if they can get past their innate differences. The strong and hearty temperament of Leo may be too much for the subtle and sensitive Pisces. Pisces, with resilience, takes on the changing moods of any partnership. While Leo is flattered by the dependency of others, Pisces may be too much for Leo to take over a long period of time.

HAPPINESS LIES IN POSITIVE LIVING
BE POSITVE THINK POSITIVE LIVE POSITIVE
CHAPTER NINTEEN
HOW TO CREATE POSITIVITY THROUGH
COMPATABILITY OF ZODIAC SIGNS
VIRGO WITH OTHER ZODIAC SIGNS
VIRGO WITH ARIES

Virgo is ruled by Mercury and Aries is ruled by Mars. But they have totally different ideas. Aries's passions are impulsive and direct. Virgo's sexuality is more enigmatic and takes time to be revealed. In other areas Aries is full of exciting new plans and ideas, and insists on being boss. Virgo is critical and fussy, and likes things to be done the way he wants. They end up making war, not love and do not blend well astrologically. Virgos desire a well-ordered existence and won't be happy under Arian leadership. If the Arian allows Virgo space, and acknowledges the virtues of Virgo, the two can make for a dynamic relationship.

VIRGO WITH TAURUS

With both being earth signs there will be much common ground for these two. Both Virgo and Taurus desire material success and security. Taurus keeps a careful eye on expenditures, which pleases Virgo. Although they lack what might be called a spontaneous approach to life, neither puts a high value on that. Both share the same intellectual pursuits. Taurus's attraction and Virgo's sharp mind are a good combination for success as a team. The one drawback is that Virgo is normally in control of their emotional output while Taurus thrives on deep emotion and could perhaps overwhelm Virgo.

VIRGO WITH GEMINI

Both are Mercury-ruled and have a mental approach to life. They are attracted to each other because of a mutual interest in intellectual ideas. Both have active minds. Virgo's analytical approach seems like indifference to Gemini. Virgo looks on Gemini's busy social life as superficial and a waste of time. Virgo is critical; Gemini is tactless. Mercury is calculating and logical; in Virgo it is critical and demanding. Gemini's ever-present desire for change would be much for the realistic Virgo. One point for the two to be compatible would be the desire for good clothes, cleanliness, mutual desire for friends and associates who are engaged in intellectual and artistic pursuits. Gemini can deal with Virgo's critical eye, well, this could work.

VIRGO WITH CANCER

Virgo's demands may be a bit much for Cancer's desire for peace and quiet. Cancer's response is emotive while Virgo's is analytical. Cancer may have to warm up Virgo a little, since there is fire under the ice. This can turn into a comfortable, and affectionate relationship. Cancer's struggle for financial security works perfectly with Virgo. Cancer's dependency neatly complements Virgo's need to protect, and each is anxious to please the other.   The full, affectionate feelings of cancer will not be completely satisfied by Virgo's direct approach to the practical matters at hand. Virgo will appreciate the loyalty and sincerity of cancer, but will need to be a little more demonstrative and affectionate with cancer.

VIRGO WITH LEO

Virgo being the earth sign and Leo being a fire sign. Here is a good chance for a happy partnership. Virgo is practical Leo is extravagant and a spendthrift. Leo likes to live life in a really big way, but Virgo is conservative. This is one of those relationships that depend, n the type of relationship it is. Leo will overwhelm Virgo, whose criticism will irk Leo. In business it is best when Leo leads and Virgo follows and the differences will be tolerated. Both of them should look elsewhere. If Virgo will permit Leo to hold the limelight and refrain from being too critical they should have no real barriers to a happy and successful partnership. But this may be quite hard.

VIRGO WITH VIRGO

Since both being the earth signs their comparability speaks of their ego problems that they may be facing while adhering to each other's view. Each of them has to forgo their egos. All is smooth sailing as long as these perfectionists curb their instincts for finding fault. Actually, they bring out the very best in each other. They are responsible, sensitive, intelligent, and take love seriously. They also share passions of the mind, and will never bore each other. Important things. Finding anything resembling compatibility would be hard for this combination. Both have a tendency to end up with a battle of the wits with both opponents evenly matched. Each would over exaggerate the faults of the other.

VIRGO WITH LIBRA

Virgo is an earth sign and Libra is and air sign. Libra enjoys spending money, going to parties, and being the center of attention. Virgo will try to curb and dominate Libra's fickle and outer directed nature. Virgo is reserved and practical, and Libra views this as a personal rebuff. Libra will soon drift away in search of more fun-loving companions. Libra may tap Virgo's hidden sensuality but their personalities are altogether too different for real compatibility. Another combination that would have trouble finding a good marital life. Their understanding and their married life can come to settlement provided each of the other forgoes the individual ego.

VIRGO WITH SCORPIO

Virgo belongs to the earth sign while Scorpio belongs to the water sign. The combination sometimes belongs to the mutual admiration society. If Virgo will keep from hurting Scorpio's pride, this combination will be happy and enduring. Scorpio is also possessive and fiercely loyal, which makes Virgo feel loved and protected. They also admire each other's minds. Virgo is logical, intellectual, and analytical. Scorpio is imaginative, visionary, and perceptive. Scorpio is volatile but secretive, Virgo is self-restrained and reserved. The Virgo mind is very fascinated with the mysterious and intriguing Scorpio. The only problem here is on the emotional side. If each of them keeps their emotion aside there is some hope for a longer lasting friendship.

VIRGO WITH SAGITTARIUS

Virgo is an earth sign and Sagittarius is a fire sign. Their comparability often leads to unwanted and undesired conflicts. Though both are intellectual signs but the way their minds work clashes with each other. Sagittarius is expansive and extravagant, while Virgo prefers a simple, ordered, and unpretentious life. Sagittarius's free spirit has nothing in common with hardworking Virgo. The differences here are like day and night. Not all bad but difficult to reconcile with.

VIRGO WITH CAPRICORN

Since these are two earth signs the mercury and sun combination should find mutual grounds for an agreeable partnership. A harmonious pair. Both are diligent, disciplined, and have a sense of purpose. They admire one another and take great pride in pleasing each other. Both need respect and approval and each intuitively gives the other exactly that. With these two signs there are some similarity and compatibility. They are both very exacting. This stops many areas of disagreement. They both take great pride in appearance and surroundings. They can find a friend in each other.

VIRGO WITH AQUARIUS

Virgo is an earth sign while Aquarius is an air sign. Aquarius has venturesome ideas and thinks Virgo unresponsive or cold. A lot depends on the cultural and educational levels of the partners. Aquarius is interested in other people, causes and Virgo is cautious about emotional giving. Virgo seeks personal achievement and financial security. Aquarius is outgoing, inventive, a visionary. Virgo is reserved, prudent, and very practical about its ambitions. This couple may not even make it as friends. There is a marked difference between the two; the chances for a happy and enduring marriage are almost nil. Each has a distant quality. There is no happy medium with this combination; it is either very good or very bad.

VIRGO WITH PISCES

Pisces is fascinated by Virgo's incisive, analytical mind. Virgo, love means security and mental compatibility. Pisces is the very opposite of Virgo as opposites often are sentimental and are poles apart. It will take a great deal of patience and understanding on the part of Virgo to cope with the sentimental nature of Pisces. This is another pair of zodiac opposites that can be great at times and horrible at others times. The opposites can learn a lot about themselves from their counterparts. It will go a long way in making this combination happy.

HAPPINESS LIES IN POSITIVE LIVING
BE POSITVE THINK POSITIVE LIVE POSITIVE
CHAPTER TWENTY
HOW TO CREATE POSITIVITY THROUGH
COMPATABILITY OF ZODIAC SIGNS
LIBRA WITH OTHER ZODIAC SIGNS
LIBRA WITH ARIES

Libra being an air sign and is a fire sign. Libra wants peace, quiet, and harmony while Aries wants action and adventure. Both like social life, entertaining, and pleasure, but both are restless in their ways. There is a powerful initial attraction between these two but their love life may be bit unconventional. Libra will look for someone less demanding, and Aries will bind someone for more dictating. Marvelous affair but poor marriage shows. Libra's refined and artistic temperament wishes for reciprocal attachments. And this is something Aries cannot provide. There is a wider the ordinary margin for error though, and most of these combinations will go at the distance and nonreciprocal.

LIBRA WITH TAURUS

Libra an air sign loves to roam and Taurus an earth sign loves to sit and waits patiently. With understanding it could be a harmonic relationship. Taurus balances Libra's indecisiveness. Taurus finds Libra a warm, romantic, partner. Libra is born to charm. The love goddess and it does shine on the two lovebirds that are until one-steps out of line. Both signs are ruled by Venus and have sensual natures, but each expresses this quality differently. However there are common interest and a meeting of the mind and body making this a very good marital combination. They appreciate beauty and the finer things of life.

LIBRA WITH GEMINI

These two air signs are well suited in every way. Both signs have much in common and enough to make an ideal partnership. Libra being under Venus's influence and Mercury ruling Gemini makes for a very good planetary combination. This will be a very stimulating relationship. One sign compliments the other and brings out the better part of each other's nature. Gemini will find it easy to communicate with Libra who is only too happy to share his information and ideas. They are affectionate, fun loving, entertaining, and travel fond. This is considered to be a great astrological influence for a long and happy marriage.

LIBRA WITH CANCER

Cancer is not temperamentally suited to cope with the freedom loving Libran. This pair operates on entirely different levels. Cancer is too temperamental and possessive for airy Libra. They both love a beautiful home, but Libra also needs parties and people and outside pleasures. When Cancer turns critical, especially about Libra's extravagance, Libra starts looking elsewhere. On the positive side though, they could make it. Ruled by the Moon and Venus respectively, there is common ground here despite the fact that we have a water sign and an air. Libra will appreciate Cancer's loyalty and generosity. Cancer wants love Libra seeks perfect intellectual communion.

LIBRA WITH LEO

Leo being a fire and Libra being an air sign. The comparability of this two shall be tiring affair. The hale and hearty Leo may prove to be too much for the sensitive Libra nature, though they have a lot in common that could make for a good combination. The sun ruling Leo and Venus ruling Libra usually form a strong and luxurious aspect. Libra is indecisive and Leo will naturally take charge. Both signs love luxuries, are subject to flattery, and are very artistically inclined. The book may not always balance because they're both extravagant and love a beautiful setting in which to shine. Each will also try to outdo the other in order to get attention.

LIBRA WITH VIRGO

Libra is and air sign and Virgo is an earth sign Libra enjoys spending money, going to parties, and being the center of attention. Virgo will try to curb and dominate Libra's fickle and outer directed nature. Virgo is reserved and practical, and Libra views this as a personal rebuff. Libra will soon drift away in search of more fun-loving companions. Libra may tap Virgo's hidden sensuality but their personalities are altogether too different for real compatibility. Another combination that would have trouble finding a good marital life. Their understanding and their married life can come to settlement provided each of the other forgoes the individual ego.

LIBRA WITH LIBRA

Whereas both are air signs. They both have basically the same interests and qualities, so there would be great understanding in the relationship. The biggest problem may be unresolved conflicts, as neither wants to stir the pot when differences appear. Equally demonstrative, lively, warm, sociable, in love with beautiful things, a problem is that neither wants to face reality. Though they are charming, peace loving, and adaptable, each needs a stronger balance than the other can provide. Also, because they are so much alike. Here is a match made in heaven, unless one had an incompatible sign rising at birth. . While both like to be admired. With this combination there is so much in common and so little negatives

LIBRA WITH SCORPIO

Libra is an air sign whereas Scorpio is a water sign. Libra may find Scorpio's intense nature a bit overwhelming. Common goals and shared interests could avert any difficulties. There is much sympathetic magnetism between these two signs. While Scorpio is the more dominating sign of the two. There is much to recommend this union, for they have many sympathies in common. Librans are sentimental and susceptible as lovers. This seems to be appealing to Scorpio's dominant and possessive urges. Scorpio is also touchy, moody, and quick to lash out in anger, which is just the kind of person Libra cannot bear. Scorpio seethes and becomes steadily more jealous and demanding, Libra has either to submit or to leave.

LIBRA WITH SAGITTARIUS

Libra being an air sign while Sagittarius being a fire sign. Their comparability is often marked by ego problems if one is able to forgo his/her ego this match can become a lasting affair. They will do well together, if Sagittarius can manage to be around enough to fulfil Libra's need for togetherness. Libra is stimulated by Sagittarius's eagerness for adventure, and Sagittarius is drawn to Libra's affectionate charm. Both are highly romantic, though this quality is more dominant in Libra. Libra will want to settle down before flighty Sagittarius does, but they can work that out. Charming, clever Libra knows how to appeal to Sagittarius's intellectual side and easily keeps Sagittarius intrigued. Sagittarius hates bondage and cannot be confined, and will not tolerate bondage, whether it be legal or not, and will use all the means at his command to break through bonds.

LIBRA WITH CAPRICORN

Libra is an air sign whereas Capricorn is an earth sign. Capricorn believes in hard work and achievement at any price. Libra is fond of socializing and nightlife, while Capricorn tends to be a loner, comfortable with only a chosen few. Libra needs flattery and attention, but Capricorn keeps its affections buried. Capricorn. And Libra's lazy, easygoing ways will offend. On the surface these two seem to be on the opposite, but the Capricorn is very much influenced by Libra. If Libra does not find the steady Capricorn nature too boring, there is good chance here for a successful marriage.

Libra had better screen the social environment to suit Capricorn's views or there may be some embarrassing moments later on. Unless Capricorn can open up a little more there could be problems here. Libra requires affection and Capricorn tends to put it off.

LIBRA WITH AQUARIUS

Since both belongs to the Air signs, their comparability can said to be lasting affair. This could be a good combination for marriage. And these two have all the makings for a beautiful friendship: harmonious vibes in socializing, artistic interests, even in involvement in public affairs. Indecisive Libra is delighted with the fact that quick-minded Aquarius likes to make decisions. Possibility one of the few problems may be a misunderstanding because an Aquarius mate is unpredictable at times, and for no reason at all, may seek seclusion and refuse to communicate. In that event, the best thing to do would be to let them enjoy their solitude. Both of these signs are naturally friendly people, while Libra is best at relationship. There may not be monumental disagreements between these two but Libra will need to understand the Aquarian perfectly.

LIBRA WITH PISCES

Libra is an air sign while Pisces is a water sign. This is a reasonably good combination. There is mutual attraction. This is especially true under intimate circumstances. Pisces will be content with Libra's exclusive company. They start off fine, since both are sentimental and affectionate. Pisces feels neglected, and whines and scolds. Pisces senses that Libra's commitment is often insincere and that Libra's charm is mostly superficial. But Libra's love of social affairs may generate jealousy and disharmony in the intimate life. Libra can get along will with nice people, but the Pisces is more discriminating, and this is the source of their disagreements. There is a mutual appreciation for art and beauty and all that it entails between these two.

HAPPINESS LIES IN POSITIVE LIVING

BE POSITVE THINK POSITIVE LIVE POSITIVE

CHAPTER TWENTY ONE

HOW TO CREATE POSITIVITY THROUGH

COMPATABILITY OF ZODIAC SIGNS

SCORPIO WITH ARIES

Whereas Scorpio being a water sign and Aries being a fire sign. With Mars dominating both signs it makes for very positive temperaments unless there are some bad natal planetary aspects. Since Aries won't take orders from Scorpions and Scorpio will never take a back seat. Love cannot be a bonfire between these two. Though they've physical, energetic, and passionate in their sexual nature and each has a forceful personality and wants to control the other there is no room for these two. This combination is can make an ideal match if one ignores to dominate the other.

SCORPIO WITH TAURUS

These two are opposites in the zodiac, but they have more in common than other opposites. Both are determined and ambitious, and neither is much of a lover. These are zodiac opposites, but they are compatible earth and water signs. This usually manifests itself in a strong physical attraction. This combination mutually admires each other. Jealousy however is the big problem with this pair and that seems to be always showing its face. Taurus must be careful to keep faith with the scorpion, or else this combination will fall down without warning.

SCORPIO WITH GEMINI

An air sign with a water sign. These two will have some difficulty rectifying their innate natures. Gemini is too changeable and inconstant for intense Scorpio, who needs and demands total commitment. Scorpio is basically a loner; Gemini likes to glitter in social settings. Gemini has a strong penchant for independence, while Scorpio wants to dominate and possess. Gemini's desire for freedom of action will clash with the jealous and possessive nature of Scorpio. These two will have some difficulty rectifying their innate natures. Then again, too much, stifles some. These two are opposites in the zodiac and are attracted to each other like magnets.

SCORPIO WITH CANCER

Both are ruled by water signs. Cancer is loyal; Scorpio's jealousy isn't provoked. Cancer admires Scorpio's strength while Scorpio finds a haven in Cancer's emotional commitment. Both are extremely intuitive and sense what will please the other. Together they can build a happy home where they feel safe and loved. This relationship has great intimacy, intensity, and depth. Things just get better all the time. Scorpio should make a good mate for quiet spoken cancer. Scorpio and cancer could well prove the ideal marriage combination.

SCORPIO WITH LEO

Leo being a fire sign and Scorpio being water sign. Two very strong willed individuals generally create some rather stormy moments. But Leo finds it hard to cope with Scorpio's jealousy and possessiveness. Scorpio considers Leo a showpiece. Scorpio doesn't understand Leo's need to be continually surrounded by an admiring audience. Scorpio would rather dominate than admire, and that doesn't suit Leo's kingly state. Two shinning personalities join together. Basically this should make for one of the most compatible combinations, but long and happy partnership will be far better a Leo female marries a Scorpio male.

SCORPIO WITH VIRGO

Virgo belongs to the earth sign while Scorpio belongs to the water sign. The combination sometimes belongs to the mutual admiration society. If Virgo will keep from hurting Scorpio's pride, this combination will be happy and enduring. Scorpio is also possessive and fiercely loyal, which makes Virgo feel loved and protected. They also admire each other's minds. Virgo is logical, intellectual, and analytical. Scorpio is imaginative, visionary, and perceptive. Scorpio is volatile but secretive, Virgo is self-restrained and reserved. The Virgo mind is very fascinated with the mysterious and intriguing Scorpio. The only problem here is on the emotional side. If each of them keeps their emotion aside there is some hope for a longer lasting friendship.

SCORPIO WITH LIBRA

Libra is an air sign whereas Scorpio is a water sign. Libra may find Scorpio's intense nature a bit overwhelming. Common goals and shared interests could avert any difficulties. There is much sympathetic magnetism between these two signs. While Scorpio is the more dominating sign of the two. There is much to recommend this union, for they have many sympathies in common. Librans are sentimental and susceptible as lovers. This seems to be appealing to Scorpio's dominant and possessive urges. As long as Libra does not hurt Scorpio's pride, Libran will find what they are looking for when they marry a Scorpio. Scorpio is also touchy, moody, and quick to lash out in anger, which is just the kind of person Libra cannot bear. Scorpio seethes and becomes steadily more jealous and demanding, Libra has either to submit-or to leave.

SCORPIO WITH SCORPIO

Since both belong to the water signs. These two people who are so much alike understand each other very little. They are highly jealous and demanding. Both are sulky, brooding, and possessive. Both are in a continual struggle to force the other to relinquish control. Where is a combination that is confusing in its outcome? If both individuals have a thorough understanding of their inherent traits, they can have deep sympathy for each other. The dominant, possessive, and jealous temperaments of each are things which both will have to handle with extreme consideration. This can be a very good combination or a very bad one.

SCORPIO WITH SAGITTARIUS

Scorpio is a water sign and Sagittarius is a fire. The combination of these to signs is an affair without proper and secured future. Scorpio is dominant by nature, but Scorpio will have trouble keeping their Sagittarian partner under control. Sagittarius is open, talkative, and casual about relationships. Scorpio wants Sagittarius at home, Sagittarius wants to roam. Mutual distrust is easy here. The Scorpion possessiveness will make life unbearable for Sagittarius. Scorpio is attractive to the

Sagittarian lust, but that is where the compatibility ends. Not a recommended combination. Live and learn is about the best thing to expect here. Both can bring out some of the other's better qualities but the chance of anything long lasting is remote.

SCORPIO WITH CAPRICORN

Scorpio belongs to a water sign and Capricorn is of earth sign. This is a very hard combination to analyse. Capricorn even likes Scorpio's jealousy-for that makes Capricorn feel secure. These two share a sense of purpose: they are ambitious, determined, and serious about responsibility-and as a team have good auguries for financial success. The emotional incompatibility usually becomes unbearable for the combination to handle. For practical matters there are common traits, but the stubborn nature of both signs could make them enemies when things get down and dirty.

SCORPIO WITH AQUARIUS

Scorpio being water sign and Aquarius being an air sign. The comparability often leads to a breaking affair. This combination usually ends up getting into unpleasant terms after a little time. Unpredictable Aquarius is too much for the solid Scorpio temperament. Aquarius has many of outside interests and this does not sit well with Scorpio. Aquarius is too reserved for the passionate Scorpio. Humanitarian instincts are what Scorpio admires in an Aquarian, but Scorpio has no interest in sharing them with the world.

Scorpio wants to possess the person and Aquarius want to own the world. Without some extremely mature attitude adjustment it will be difficult to rectify the inherent differences in each other's nature. Scorpio wants to stay at home; Aquarius wants to be free to go.

SCORPIO WITH PISCES

Everything seems fine until Pisces gets tired of the little interests that seem to keep Scorpio occupied outside of the home. Scorpio does not appreciate positive qualities of Pisces. Pisces' imagination sparks Scorpio's creativity. Pisces' intuitive awareness and Scorpio's depth of feeling unite in a special closeness. This kind of mating lasts. This may be a love at first sight combination, however it seldom lasts a long period of time. But, on the positive side there is an intuitive bond here that both will find agreeable. There is attraction and emotion and feelings and all that good stuff that they both like.

HAPPINESS LIES IN POSITIVE LIVING

BE POSITVE THINK POSITIVE LIVE POSITIVE

CHAPTER TWENTY TWO

HOW TO CREATE POSITIVITY THROUGH

COMPATABILITY OF ZODIAC SIGNS

SAGITTARIUS WITH OTHER ZODIAC SIGNS

SAGITTARIUS WITH ARIES

The Mars-Jupiter duo is usually an ideal match for each other. Sagittarius is a perfect ideal and temperamental match for Aries. They both are active, spontaneous people. There may be a little conflict because both are impulsive and brutally frank. However, they have wonderful senses of humor and enjoy each other's company. If they make it in the bedroom, they'll make it everywhere else. Most people of these matches are in it for life. The Sagittarius means liberty, and the pursuit of happiness while Aries is subscribes to this theory. And for this reason, that makes them a good match.

SAGITTARIUS WITH TAURUS

These are two very different personality types the more reserved Taurus and the outgoing Sagittarius both has an appreciation for the truth. Sagittarius has an easy live and let live attitude this might work if Taurus can tie a string to Sagittarius's. The Taurus who marries a Sagittarian will find that no amount of arguing or berating is going to change the reckless Sagittarian With some understanding they can find harmony in their characters as long as they allow each other their personalities. With the Taurean being possessive and the Sagittarian being freedom loving, the Sagittarian may find this hard to co-operate with.

SAGITTARIUS WITH GEMINI

Mercury rules Gemini and Sagittarius are ruled by Jupiter the planet of knowledge and wisdom. Both have bright minds, but Sagittarius is outspoken while Gemini likes to enjoy fun. They are usually a compatible combination with both being frank, outspoken, and a certain amount of personal understanding being made. They meet on a common ground, and can plan their lives with equilibrium. They are restless, adventuresome, imaginative, and fun loving. No other opposite signs in the zodiac enjoy each other more than these two. However if Sagittarius forgoes its ego and Gemini restores to concrete planning they can make a good combination otherwise their combination may not last long.

SAGITTARIUS WITH CANCER

A water and fire combination. Sagittarius likes to wander, while Cancer is a prefers to stay at home. Cancer's commitment to total togetherness only makes Sagittarius desperate to get away. In addition, outspoken Sagittarius's bluntness continually wounds sensitive Cancer. They happen to be better friends than lovers. There is a vast difference in natures and the likely hood of being compatible is all but impossible, unless there are some positive aspects in their charts. Cancer is too needy for Sagittarius. On the good side, they are both generous people.

SAGITTARIUS WITH LEO

Both being of fire sign. The pendulum can swing in any body's favour. Together they share a liking for freedom, adventure, and meeting new people. Leo's natural quality of leadership brings out what loyalty Sagittarius can give. Leo is very proud, but self-confident and expansive Sagittarius is quite happy to let Leo go. Both love change and excitement and have a great zest for life. This is an excellent combination for the most part unless Sagittarius is in need of too much freedom and Leo becomes too bossy.

SAGITTARIUS WITH VIRGO

Virgo is an earth sign and Sagittarius is a fire sign. Their comparability often leads to unwanted and undesired conflicts. Though both are intellectual signs but the way their minds work clashes with each other. Sagittarius is expansive and extravagant, while Virgo prefers a simple, ordered, and unpretentious life. Sagittarius's free spirit has nothing in common with hardworking Virgo. The differences here are like day and night. Not all bad but difficult to reconcile with.

SAGITTARIUS WITH LIBRA

Libra being an air signs while Sagittarius being a fire sign. Their comparability is often marked by ego problems if one is able to forgo his/her ego this match can become a lasting affair. They will do well together, if Sagittarius can manage to be around enough to fulfil Libra's need for togetherness. Libra is stimulated by Sagittarius's eagerness for adventure, and Sagittarius is drawn to Libra's affectionate charm.

 Both are highly romantic, though this quality is more dominant in Libra. Libra will want to settle down before flighty Sagittarius does, but they can work that out. Charming, clever Libra knows how to appeal to Sagittarius's intellectual side and easily keeps Sagittarius intrigued. Sagittarius hates bondage and cannot be confined, and will not tolerate bondage, whether it be legal or not, and will use all the means at his command to break through bonds.

SAGITTARIUS WITH SCORPIO

Scorpio is a water sign and Sagittarius is a fire. The combination of these to signs is an affair without proper and secured future. Scorpio is dominant by nature, but Scorpio will have trouble keeping their Sagittarian partner under control. Sagittarius is open, talkative, and casual about relationships. Scorpio wants Sagittarius at home, Sagittarius wants to roam. Mutual distrust is easy here. The Scorpion possessiveness will make life unbearable for Sagittarius. Scorpio is attractive to the Sagittarian lust, but that is where the compatibility ends. Not a recommended combination. Live and learn is about the best thing to expect here. Both can bring out some of the other's better qualities but the chance of anything long lasting is remote.

SAGITTARIUS WITH SAGITTARIUS

Since both belong to fire signs. Their combination would be a sweet- sour affair. Two lively, optimistic people on the go all the time. But this exciting, chaotic, eventful relationship is too unpredictable to suit either of them. They have a tendency to bring out the worst in each other. Each remains uncommitted and has so many outside interests that this pair inevitably drifts apart. If this combination is not on the same intellectual and social plane, there is little hope for this couple to have a long happy relationship. They will have to do everything together or nothing at all. All interests being social and business must be the same. May work better as friends or partners.

SAGITTARIUS WITH CAPRICORN

Sagittarius belongs to a fire sign whereas Capricorn attributes to earth sign. Sagittarius is venturesome, sociable, and expansive.

Capricorn is cautious with money and concerned with appearances and Sagittarius is neither. Both should look elsewhere. Capricorn and the outgoing, risk taking Sagittarius. Not much in the way of compatibility but as with most combinations they can learn from each other. Sagittarius may prove to be too much for the sombre and restrictive temperament of Capricorn. Their temperament is entirely different, one is optimistic, and the other is pessimistic. Here again we see the difference between them may not be a lasting affair.

SAGITTARIUS WITH AQUARIUS

Sagittarius is a fire sign whereas Aquarius is an air sign. Their comparability often results in a powerful combination. Each of the other has to forgo his or her own ego. Aquarius is innovative. Sagittarius loves to experiment. These two share a great zest for living and a forward-looking viewpoint. Neither will try to tie down the other. Both seek to explore possibilities to the fullest, and they share idealism about love and life. They'll like each other too. The combination usually has a great chance for success. Both temperaments are very much alike. This is a purely social combination that will revel in a large group of friends and public-spirited associates. Sagittarius readily understands the moods and peculiarities of the Aquarius. There is a very good chance for a successful relationship.

SAGITTARIUS WITH PISCES

Sagittarius is a fire sign and Pisces is water. There is much here for an interesting and sincere relationship. Sagittarius is attracted to Pisces's spirituality. Sagittarius being free and easy will find Pisces too much of a heavy load to haul around. Though, Sagittarius may find that the marriage to Pisces is too confining. There will be a lot of confusion and wonder between these two. At times it will be good and at other times not good at all. Your natures are somewhat opposite to one another and the ability to understand the other's intent and actions will be evident. This combination quite hard to match.

HAPPINESS LIES IN POSITIVE LIVING
BE POSITVE THINK POSITIVE LIVE POSITIVE
CHAPTER TWENTY THREE
HOW TO CREATE POSITIVITY THROUGH
COMPATABILITY OF ZODIAC SIGNS
CAPRICORN WITH OTHER ZODIAC SIGNS
CAPRICORN WITH ARIES

Capricorns are usually patient and are traditionally easygoing. Arians are too impatient to cope with the slowness attitude. Saturn represents the Capricorn and Mars governs the Aries. Aries's taste for innovation and experiment may not please Capricorns. Aries is restless, fiery, and impulsive; Capricorn is ordered, settled, and practical. Capricorn needs to dominate and so does Aries. Problems often crops up over moneymaking schemes. Not a hopeful combination. Capricorn will nod against the Arian will and a disagreement is bound to occur. In the matter of sex there is an affinity; however, their inherent personalities clash. The combination of a fire sign with an earth sign. Aries is a fiery in nature while Capricorn is earth, cautious and reserved. Aries prefers to take action while Capricorn would rather plan and wait. Without a great deal of tolerance and patience, there is not much hope for this union.

CAPRICORN WITH TAURUS

A good combination of the basic earth signs. Both are responsible and practical natures. They even have a mutual desire for success and material things. Capricorn is a strong match for Taurus, for they both have passions that are straightforward and uncomplicated. Capricorn is a bit more secretive than Taurus. With both partners having mutual understanding of each other's personalities this can be a very compatible marriage. Venus and Saturn blend very well from an emotional point of view.

CAPRICORN WITH GEMINI

Capricorn gets worried about security, while Gemini feels about losing its liberty. The Saturn ruled Capricorn will be at differences with the Mercury ruled Gemini. Patience is a virtue with Capricorn, but it is not so with Gemini. Gemini's need for a survival does nothing to make Capricorn feel secure. Gemini's free talks, meets opposition from conservative Capricorn. Capricorn's great drive to execute will prove to be too much for the Gemini. Until they both are ready to minimize their goals. Capricorn will go on hunting until he gains the upper hand. Of course with these two people going together anything is possible and the outcome of the result may not be satisfying to each other.

CAPRICORN WITH CANCER

Both signs have plenty in common. Capricorn has too many other interests to give Cancer all the attention it needs. Cancer is shy, sensitive, and needs affection, while Capricorn is aloof, and domineering. Capricorn has the ability to make cancer's dream come true, while Cancer is happy wishing for and wanting the success and security that the Capricorn strives for. The elements of water and earth go well together but these are zodiac opposites you can expect both side of the coin. They will have to take the good with the bad and there will be plenty of both. Capricorn lacks the warmth and sentiment that Cancer requires.

CAPRICORN WITH LEO

Leo being a fire signs whereas Capricorn is an earth sign. The combination of these two may at time lead to severe complications. The slow Capricorn may prove to be too much for the carefree nature of Leo. Leo will think Capricorn stingy with affection because Capricorn's reserved, undemonstrative nature cannot give Leo the adoration it needs. Neither will take a back seat nor let the other dominate. This affair will be on the rocks before it even leaves the dock. Leo forgives and forgets; Capricorn being the one who is slow to anger and seldom forgets. This pair would not form the ideal basis for mutual understanding. Leo likes to live for the moment and Capricorn prefers to make calculated movements.

CAPRICORN WITH VIRGO

Since these are two earth signs the mercury and sun combination should find mutual grounds for an agreeable partnership. A harmonious pair. Both are diligent, disciplined, and have a sense of purpose. They admire one another and take great pride in pleasing each other. Both need respect and approval and each intuitively gives the other exactly that. With these two signs there are some similarity and compatibility. They are both very exacting. This stops many areas of disagreement. They both take great pride in appearance and surroundings.

CAPRICORN WITH LIBRA

Libra is an air sign whereas Capricorn is an earth sign. Capricorn believes in hard work and achievement at any price. Libra is fond of socializing and nightlife, while Capricorn tends to be a loner, comfortable with only a chosen few. Libra needs flattery and attention, but Capricorn keeps its affections buried. Capricorn.

And Libra's lazy, easygoing ways will offend. On the surface these two seem to be on the opposite, but the Capricorn is very much influenced by Libra. If Libra does not find the steady Capricorn nature too boring, there is good chance here for a successful marriage. Libra had better screen the social environment to suit Capricorn's views or there may be some embarrassing moments later on. Unless Capricorn can open up a little more there could be problems here. Libra requires affection and Capricorn tends to put it off.

CAPRICORN WITH SCORPIO

Scorpio belongs to a water sign and Capricorn is of earth sign. This is a very hard combination to analyse. Capricorn even likes Scorpio's jealousy-for that makes Capricorn feel secure. These two share a sense of purpose: they are ambitious, determined, and serious about responsibility-and as a team have good auguries for financial success. The emotional incompatibility usually becomes unbearable for the combination to handle. For practical matters there are common traits, but the stubborn nature of both signs could make them enemies when things get down and dirty.

CAPRICORN WITH SAGITTARIUS

Sagittarius belongs to a fire sign whereas Capricorn attributes to earth sign. Sagittarius is venturesome, sociable, and expansive. Capricorn is cautious with money and concerned with appearances and Sagittarius is neither. Both should look elsewhere. Capricorn and the outgoing, risk taking Sagittarius. Not much in the way of compatibility but as with most combinations they can learn from each other. Sagittarius may prove to be too much for the somber and restrictive temperament of Capricorn. Their temperament is entirely different, one is optimistic, and the other is pessimistic. Here again we see the difference between them may not be a lasting affair.

CAPRICORN WITH CAPRICORN

Both belong to earth sign. They both have the same faults, which may keep fault finding down to a minimum. With important issues, they would both have what it takes to over come any hardship. Capricorns approve of people like themselves, so with these two there's no lack of mutual respect and regard. Neither one can relax or let down its hair. Both have the same long-range aspirations and the basic qualities to attain them. Great mixture for a happy relationship. The biggest problem here will be keeping things lively and new.

CAPRICORN WITH AQUARIUS

Since Capricorn being an earth sign and Aquarius being an air sign Capricorn believes in self-discipline and Aquarius believes in self-expression. Capricorn finds Aquarius too unpredictable, and Aquarius's impersonal attitude makes Capricorn uneasy. However, they should like each other and love can turn into friendship. This is a very hard combination to analyse. Capricorn wants all effort and anything else Aquarius has to give- to be cantered at home for their mutual good. Capricorn does not like the interest that Aquarius shows to other people. A very doubtful combination. Too many other differences as well and unless you have other compatible aspects in your birth charts, don't expect a long lasting affair.

CAPRICORN WITH PISCES

As Capricorn being an earth sign and Pisces being a water sign. This is a good combination with complimentary values. And there's nothing Capricorn likes better than being admired. Pisces generous affections and Capricorn's strong sense of loyalty combine to make each feel safe and protected. These very different people meet each other's needs. One of the things that Pisces will admire about Capricorn is his very practical ways.

HAPPINESS LIES IN POSITIVE LIVING
BE POSITVE THINK POSITIVE LIVE POSITIVE
CHAPTER TWENTY FOUR
HOW TO CREATE POSITIVITY THROUGH COMPATABILITY OF ZODIAC SIGNS
COMPATABILITY
ZODIAC SIGNS
AQUARIUS WITH OTHER ZODIAC SIGNS

Aquarius belongs to an air sign whereas Aries belongs to fire sign. Both signs are of independent nature but at times Aquarius will do things without notice with which Aries may become impatient. Since both are active, ambitious, enjoy a wide range of interests, and are equally eager for sexual adventure. As both are independent Aquarius energies more than Aries and Aries may at times feel neglected. Aries finds the Aquarian unpredictability exciting, but feels entirely insecure. However, with a bit of tact and understanding on both sides, this is a great affair that could turn into something even better. This could possibly be a good relationship, but will require a positive attitude on both parts.

AQUARIUS WITH TAURUS

These two live on opposite sides of the planet, in fact sometimes, Taurus will wonder if Aquarius is even from this planet. Neither is likely to approve of the other. Taurus is conservative, careful, closemouthed. Aquarius is unconventional, innovative, and vivacious. Taurus is lusty and passionate while Taurus needs security and comfort. Aquarius, a fancy-free loner who resents ties that bind. This combination heads in for many difficulties. The Aquarian being unpredictable. Both love ease and comfort but their views on how to obtain them are very different. Another big irritation for the Taurus lover is the unwillingness of the Aquarius to share his secrets. Aquarius will find the Taurus attention somewhat smothering and restrictive

AQUARIUS WITH GEMINI

Gemini is bit inconstant or unstable, Aquarius understands somewhat Gemini's needs. Gemini is always looking for surprises and the Aquarian can give them. Gemini and Aquarius get along quite easily. They share a taste for new things, travelling, meeting new people and doing new things. Since both are unpredictable, things may always go smoothly with them. But love keeps getting them together, for Aquarius adores Gemini's wit and good cheer. The caring, thoughts of Aquarius will find a smooth home with Gemini. Uranus, the ruling planet of Aquarius, is full of surprises and sudden changes. This will suit the Gemini perfectly. There will be plenty of none stop variety to afford the stimulation that Gemini needs for its dual personality and goal.

AQUARIUS WITH CANCER

Aquarius is quick-minded, unpredictable, and apt to be impatient with cautious, hesitant Cancer. Cancer has a conservative taste while Aquarius taste is usually the opposite. Cancer needs to feel close and secure. The social side of the Aquarian may prove to be too much for the Cancer. Aquarian's love to share their life stories with the world while cancer is satisfied to concentrate on personal obligations. Odds against this combination are too great for this combination, unless one will become convergent to the other. Aquarius has a need to be independent and often appears detached in a close relationship with cancer.

AQUARIUS WITH LEO

Aquarius is an air sign and Leo is a fire sign. The comparability of this two in terms of worldly affairs can often become difficult to match. Both like socializing and meeting new people, but Leo always needs to perform on center stage, which makes Aquarius impatient and irritable. Aquarius is too independent to become Leo's devoted subject. And that's where it ends. Leo views Aquarius's aloof emotions as a personal rejection. Both signs are better when doing things for others. Leo loves the world and Aquarius loves humanity. This makes for an excellent combination for a partnership that deals with or caters to the public. Each has a mutual understanding of the other when it comes to intimate matters, needs and desires.

AQUARIUS WITH VIRGO

Aquarius is an air sign while Virgo is an earth sign. Aquarius has venturesome ideas and thinks Virgo unresponsive or cold. A lot depends on the cultural and educational levels of the partners. Aquarius is interested in other people, causes and Virgo is cautious about emotional giving. Virgo seeks personal achievement and financial security. Aquarius is outgoing, inventive, a visionary. Virgo is reserved, prudent, and very practical about its ambitions. This couple may not even make it as friends. There is a marked difference between the two; the chances for a happy and enduring marriage are almost nil.

Each has a distant quality. There is no happy medium with this combination; it is either very good or very bad.

AQUARIUS WITH LIBRA

Whereas both are air signs. They both have basically the same interests and qualities, so there would be great understanding in the relationship. The biggest problem may be unresolved conflicts, as neither wants to stir the pot when differences appear. Equally demonstrative, lively, warm, sociable, in love with beautiful things, a problem is that neither wants to face reality. Though they are charming, peace loving, and adaptable, each needs a stronger balance than the other can provide. Also, because they are so much alike. Here is a match made in heaven, unless one had an incompatible sign rising at birth. . While both likes to be admired. With this combination there is so much in common and so little negatives

AQUARIUS WITH SCORPIO

Aquarius being an air sign and Scorpio being water sign. The comparability often leads to a breaking affair. This combination usually ends up getting into unpleasant terms after a little time. Unpredictable Aquarius is too much for the solid Scorpio temperament. Aquarius has many of outside interests and this does not sit well with Scorpio. Aquarius is too reserved for the passionate Scorpio. Humanitarian instincts are what Scorpio admires in an Aquarian, but

Scorpio has no interest in sharing them with the world. Scorpio wants to possess the person and Aquarius want to own the world. Without some extremely mature attitude adjustment it will be difficult to rectify the inherent differences in each other's nature. Scorpio wants to stay at home; Aquarius wants to be free to go.

AQUARIUS WITH SAGITTARIUS

Aquarius is an air sign where as Sagittarius is a fire sign. Their comparability often results in a powerful combination. Each of the other has to forgo his or her own ego. Aquarius is innovative. Sagittarius loves to experiment. These two share a great zest for living and a forward-looking viewpoint. Neither will try to tie down the other. Both seek to explore possibilities to the fullest, and they share idealism about love and life. They'll like each other too. The combination usually has a great chance for success. Both temperaments are very much alike. This is a purely social combination that will revel in a large group of friends and public-spirited associates. Sagittarius readily understands the moods and peculiarities of the Aquarius. There is a very good chance for a successful relationship.

AQUARIUS WITH CAPRICORN

Aquarius being an air sign and Capricorn being an earth sign. Capricorn believes in self-discipline and Aquarius believes in self-expression. Capricorn finds Aquarius too unpredictable, and Aquarius's impersonal attitude makes Capricorn uneasy. However, they should like each other and love can turn into friendship. This is a very hard combination to analyse. Capricorn wants all effort and anything else Aquarius has to give- to be cantered at home for their mutual good. Capricorn does not like the interest that Aquarius shows to other people. A very doubtful combination. Too many other differences as well and unless you have other compatible aspects in your birth charts, don't expect a long lasting affair.

AQUARIUS WITH AQUARIUS

Both being an air signs. This combination is more compatible then any other combination. One Aquarius finally finds just the right mate in the other Aquarian. They admire and like each other, and especially enjoy each other's sense of humor. Each is involved in all kinds of projects and friendships. With so many outside activities going, they are likely to be apart as much as they are together and that's fine with them. They haven't a thing to quarrel about since they agree on everything: Both of them are much more rational than emotional.

AQUARIUS WITH PISCES

Aquarius is an air sign where as Pisces is a water sign. Their comparability often leads to an unconventional relationship. Pisces needs someone strong to take control. Aquarius shuns any kind of emotional demands. This can be a dreamy affair as someone should show the reality to these people and that's not to say that they are unaware of reality. Both operate in a different manner than the other signs.

If the Pisces is able give the Aquarius the benefit of the doubt, the marriage should be a lasting one.

HAPPINESS LIES IN POSITIVE LIVING
BE POSITVE THINK POSITIVE LIVE POSITIVE

CHAPTER TWENTY FIVE

HOW TO CREATE POSITIVITY THROUGH COMPATABILITY OF ZODIAC SIGNS

PISCES WITH OTHER ZODIAC SIGNS

PISCES WITH ARIES

Pisceans are romantic and they desire the delicate approach that which the Arian lacks. Aries will draw Pisces out of their shell, and in turn will be appealed by Pisces mysterious nature in terms of sexuality. The boldness and confidence of Aries adding to the Pisces's intuitions and fantasies end in an eventful union. Pisces is somewhat shy and Aries likes to be dominant, Pisces likes having someone to be looked upon. For a happy coupling thus requires only a little more tact on Arian part.

PISCES WITH TAURUS

These two can share a great deal of their appreciation for beauty, art, and sensuality and just about any of the finer things in life. Pisces may not altogether understand Taurus's materialistic approach to life. Taurus's practical, easygoing nature helps Pisces through its frequent changes of mood. In love, Taurus is devoted and Pisces adores. This usually is a very happy combination. Pisces being romantic, imaginative, impressionable and flexible is just what the Taurus native is looking for.

PISCES WITH GEMINI

Their passion is quite high, and so are their problems. Thoughtless Gemini easily hurts Pisces. Gemini is mischievous and playful, but Pisces is sensitive and takes things to heart easily. Each practices in his or her thoughts in their own way: Gemini needs freedom and Pisces needs unending appreciation. Pisces just can't feel secure with talkative moods of Gemini, and he tries to pull the net in his own way. This atmosphere eventually makes it hard for Gemini to breathe his own liberty. The freedom of Gemini is stake if he marries a Piscean. Gemini's should be prepared to change their ways if they want to seek happiness with a loving and possessive Piscean.

PISCES WITH CANCER

The water signs rule a harmonious match and quite a perfect match as both. The sentimental combination of these two signs makes for an ideal marriage. Although both will have their moments of gloom and doom, they will soon come out in the sunshine to forgive and forget each other. They are both romantic, need to love and be loved and can probably communicate to each other without speaking or making facial gestures. Both are emotional, intensely devoted, and sensitive to each other's moods.

PISCES WITH LEO

A fire and water combination. Leo being a fire sign and Pisces being a water sign often makes this a unique combination.   Both are more inclined to take than to give. Fiery Leo and watery Pisces.

This is the depiction of these two. Generally not expected to work but both have an ability to learn from one another if they can get past their innate differences. The strong and hearty temperament of Leo may be too much for the subtle and sensitive Pisces. Pisces, with resilience, takes on the changing moods of any partnership. While Leo is flattered by the dependency of others. Pisces may be too much for Leo to take over a long period of time.

PISCES WITH VIRGO

Pisces is fascinated by Virgo's incisive, analytical mind. Virgo, love means security and mental compatibility.

Pisces is the very opposite of Virgo as opposites often are sentimental and are poles apart. It will take a great deal of patience and understanding on the part of Virgo to cope with the sentimental nature of Pisces. This is another pair of zodiac opposites that can be great at times and horrible at others times. The opposites can learn a lot about themselves from their counterparts. It will go a long way in making this combination happy

PISCES WITH LIBRA

Libra is an air sign while Pisces is a water sign. This is a reasonably good combination. There is mutual attraction. This is especially true under intimate circumstances. Pisces will be content with Libra's exclusive company. They start off fine, since both are sentimental and affectionate. Pisces feels neglected, and whines and scolds. Pisces senses that Libra's commitment is often insincere and that Libra's charm is mostly superficial. But Libra's love of social affairs may generate jealousy and disharmony in the intimate life. Libra can get along will with nice people, but the Pisces is more discriminating, and this is the source of their disagreements. There is a mutual appreciation for art and beauty and all that it entails between these two.

PISCES WITH SCORPIO

Everything seems fine until Pisces gets tired of the little interests that seem to keep Scorpio occupied outside of the home. Scorpio does not appreciate positive qualities of Pisces. Pisces' imagination sparks Scorpio's creativity. Pisces' intuitive awareness and Scorpio's depth of feeling unite in a special closeness. This kind of mating lasts. This may be a love at first sight combination, however it seldom lasts a long period of time. But, on the positive side there is an intuitive bond here that both will find agreeable. There is attraction and emotion and feelings and all that good stuff that they both like.

PISCES WITH SAGITTARIUS

Sagittarius is a fire sign and Pisces is a water Sign. There is much here for an interesting and sincere relationship. Sagittarius is attracted to Pisces's spirituality. Sagittarius being free and easy will find Pisces too much of a heavy load to haul around. Though Sagittarius may find that the marriage to Pisces is too confining. There will be a lot of confusion and wonder between these two. At times it will be good and at other times not good at all. Your natures are somewhat opposite to one another and the ability to understand the other's intent and actions will be evident.

PISCES WITH CAPRICORN

As Capricorn being an earth sign and Pisces being Water sign. This is a good combination with complimentary values. And there's nothing Capricorn likes better than being admired. Pisces generous affections and Capricorn's strong sense of loyalty combine to make each feel safe and protected. These very different people meet each other's needs. One of the things that Pisces will admire about Capricorn is his very practical ways. This combination seems to work very well, provided each other admires the other's values first.

PISCES WITH AQUARIUS

Both being an Air Sign. This combination is more compatible then any other combination. One Aquarius finally finds just the right mate in the other Aquarian. They admire and like each other, and especially enjoy each other's sense of humour. Each is involved in all kinds of projects and friendships. With so many outside activities going, they are likely to be apart as much as they are together and that's fine with them. They haven't a thing to quarrel about since they agree on everything. Both of them are much more rational than emotional.

PISCES WITH PISCES

Since both belong to water sign, having the same virtues and vices they should get along well together, at least they will have understanding and sympathy for one another. They find it hard to cope with practical realities, and there's no strong partner around to push either one in the right direction. Both have the same interests and the same love of home and possessions. At least both can be anchored to each other, so that they can put their shoulders to the wheel and face the responsibilities that reality demands. They have the refinement and delicacy that each desires. This should be a good combination.

HAPPINESS LIES IN POSITIVE LIVING
BE POSITVE THINK POSITIVE LIVE POSITIVE
CHAPTER TWENTY SIX

HOW TO CREATE POSITIVITY

Thought which are provoking our mind, about the uncertainties and the negativities, as to what will happen tomorrow. Worries that are prevailing in our minds are repetitive thoughts associated with feelings of anxiety in anticipation of some negative future event. Whether the worries are about financial crisis, family problems, work, health or any topic of concern, the anxious feelings produced and sustained by the imaginary thoughts which always distinctly appear to be unpleasant. Worrying will carry tomorrow's load with today's strength. Worry will not empty tomorrow of its sorrows, it empties today of its power and strength. Worries make you to move into tomorrow ahead of time. Half the worry in the world is caused by people trying to make decisions before they have sufficient knowledge on which to base a decision. Why worry about the future. Just imagine as to what if we just acted like everything was easy and there was nothing very serious about it to come in future. Worry often gives a small thing a big shadow and its surrounding do frightened with more scary things. Why worry about tomorrow; concentrate on today happening as for tomorrow will worry about itself. Each day has its own worries and troubles. If there is not any solution to the some problem then do not waste time worrying about it. And if there is a solution to the problem then why waste time worrying about it. Worry will never rob tomorrow of its sorrows, but will only deny today of its meaning happiness and joys. Worrying is actually a form of superstition and creates false images in our mind and that is the main reason and cause which makes and leads us to this point of imagination. A human being can survive almost anything, as long as he or she sees the end in sight. If something bad or good is to happen it is sure to happen, whether we worry or not. Let us put our energy into today and stop worrying about the future and past. We should not foresee trouble, or worry about what may never happen as past is dead and gone forever and future is uncertain and yet to come. The basic facts we should know about worry. The basic techniques to analyze worry and how to break the worry habit before it breaks us. These are the simple ways where we can concentrate and get rid of worries prevailing in our thoughts .Annalise worry to see and get the reasons and facts of worry. To avoid reoccurrence of worries, concentrate on prayers as prayers are the best source of remedies of the prevailing worries. The more you pray, the less you'll panic. The more you worship, the less you worry. There is nothing that wastes the body like worry, and anyone who has any faith in God should need not to worry about anything whatsoever is to happen in future.

We ought to know the basic fundamental of analyzing worries. Worries create unnecessary thoughts and these are caused by people going in for unwanted decisions, fore hand not even knowing as to when a good decision is made and not even having sufficient knowledge about it. We must first study and after carefully weighing all the facts than only come to a powerful decision. Simply making castles in the air won't solve our problems but add more to our vows.Anxiety and worry can go hand in hand. When anxiety grabs the mind, it is self-perpetuating. Your mind gets clogged with numerous with buts and ifs. Do not worry about your life. Worries are repetitive thoughts associated with feelings of anxiety in anticipation of some negative future event. Yet anxious feelings and the worries that lead to them can prove helpful. It becomes a difficult problem if you are constantly anxious as it will become a hindrance to your everyday life, rather than motivate you to some good and better things. Never worry alone. Worrisome thoughts reproduce faster so one of the most powerful ways to stop the spiral of worry is simply to disclose the worry to a friend. What you will eat or drink; or about your body, what you will wear. If you know that the circumstance is beyond your control or power change than revise it to your liking. Just try to put a stop-less order on your worries. Don't permit little things which become insects of life to ruin your happiness. Co-operate with the inevitable. Decide just how much anxiety a thing may be worth and refuse to give in anymore. All the happiness is not given in one go it comes slowly and slowly.

If your worries center around, an important relationship in your life, pay special attention to remain positive and be happy. To keep yourself happy, treat your worried thoughts as valuable signals. How to keep from worrying about criticism? Simply unjust criticism is often a disguised compliment. It often means that you have aroused jealousy and envy. Let's keep a record of the fool things we have done and criticize ourselves.The utmost cause of worry is your state of depression. Worries are there to motivate information-gathering and problem-solving. Depression is the inability to construct a future. Depression is inertia. That's the thing about depression: But depression is so insidious, and it compounds daily, that it's impossible to ever see the end. Depressed people think they know themselves, but maybe they only know depression.

There are no hopeless than this to get depressed. Our attitude towards suffering and depression becomes very important because it can affect how we cope with suffering when it arises. Depression is nourished by a lifetime of un grieved and unforgiven causes. Never worry about your heart till it stops beating. How can you deal with anxiety? You might try what when you did. A person worried so much that he decided to hire someone to do his worrying for him. Times will change for the better when you change. Worry is a misuse of the imagination. Worry is most often a prideful way of thinking that you have more control over life and its circumstances than you actually do. To keep yourself happy, treat your worried thoughts as valuable signals. These are the fundamental facts you should be familiar about worries. A huge factor to stay happy is to cater your worries around, an important relationship in your life and pay special attention sustaining positive relationships. Worries are there to motivate information gathering and problem-solving. Make your mind firm and do come to a positive decision as come what we will not allow the worries to entire our mind and soul. Once a decision is carefully reached we should get busy carrying out our decisions and should not bother about all the anxieties that are about to come. When we, or any of our colleagues or associates, are about to worry about a problem, we must write it out and think of the following questions: Instead of worrying about what people say of you, why not spend time trying to accomplish something they will admire. What if we just acted like everything was easy? How would your life be different if you stopped worrying about things we can't control and started focusing on the things we can? Let today be the day. You free yourself from fruitless worry, seize the day and take effective action on things you can change...

HAPPINESS LIES IN POSITIVE LIVING

BE POSITVE THINK POSITIVE LIVE POSITIVE

CHAPTER TWENTY SEVEN

WHAT DO YOU GET OUTOF BEING NEGATIVE?

You may feel largely uncomfortable, when worries attack your thoughts and mind which makes worrying about a situation an easier option to get depressed and diffused. While you are consuming more worries you are far too busy to do anything else to fix the real problem and would rather find it hard to get into a smart solution. Thus resulting in a fact that you spend your evenings worrying only without even bothering to find some time to search a new job. You get nothing out of worrying except only to think and cry. Another cause of getting worried is the attachment with which your inner soul gets attracted to. Attachment brings worry. If you have a problem and you come up with the answer, you stop worrying immediately. Our minds can be dishonest, persuading us that we are worrying about something, when our deepest fear is entirely different. No-one likes to admit that they've chosen to worry. The first step is to write down your worries, which will help you make sense of them, and then decide on one small step you can take towards a solution. But to be very true no man in this world is free of obstacles or difficulties. Don't make worry your habit. Break this habit and stop all the negative and panic thoughts provoking your mind all the time.If you can't change the past, but you must not ruin the present by worrying about the future. Joy is what happens to us when we allow ourselves to recognize how good things really are. When we feel worried and depressed, we need to consciously form a smile on our faces and act upbeat until the happy feeling becomes genuine reality. Feelings of depression and hopelessness and or anger are even tougher to cope with on a consistent basis. When you are worried, you not only hurt yourself, but the limited support systems that are still holding on your mind but making you to get more and more worried and nothing is achieved in terms of success except the re-carnation of worries and worriesYour actions breed confidence and courage. If you want to conquer fear, anger and worry do not sit ideal and just think about it. Let our deep worrying become advance thinking and planning. If you look into your own mind and heart, and you find nothing wrong there, what is there to worry about? Practically nothing what is there to fear about and again nothing? So why worry unnecessarily and make your present and future dark.Why being a negative person and what do you get out of it being a depression dejected and sad man.? Why not turn your thoughts to be a positive person simply it is a question of tilting your mind towards a positive side of thing. See both the aspects of a situation and ways the pros and cons of both the sides and try to abolish the negativity in you. Think of the best the best is sure to happen and if you think of the worst the worst will come. Better come forward wake up and think positive first. Positive persons always succeed in life whatever be the circumstances and the negative often dig a death trap for themselves. So why be a negative person why you have all the qualities of being a positive man.

HAPPINESS LIES IN POSITIVE LIVING
BE POSITVE THINK POSITIVE LIVE POSITIVE
CHAPTER TWENTY EIGHT
CREATE HAPPINESS WITHIN YOU

If you are interested in getting more happiness, focus on all the ways as if you have already attained success. You need to focus on the thing and create a live within you. If you want love and affection, focus on all the people and the abundance of love that you have to give to them. If we want to have greater health, focus on all the ways that we are healthy, thus creating and delivering a good life within you. You need to admit that there are problems that you cannot change. But you can change the way of your thinking if you identify the main reason of the problem. And if you acknowledge the facts, that you have been negative or inactive in finding a solution to the problem, probably this will make it easier for you to become positive thus creating a new lease of life within you. You must try to make goals. Making goals can give you a more positive outlook on life. People often tend to get bored with life and get the feeling that they are stuck to negative things which the result they often get the feeling of being depressed. Setting a direction for yourself and a goal would surely help you to move forward. If you expecting to succeed, and are not afraid of failure, you have the best chance of staying positive and can create a very positive life within you. When you, or any of your associates, are tempted to worry about a problem, write out the solution and a definite answer to it. This helps a positive feeling to generate within you.Another thing you need to understand is that there are several ways to cultivate a mental attitude that can bring you peace and happiness and can carnage a good life within you. More of it if you fill your mind with thoughts of peace, courage, health, and hope, your life will be easy to live. You would get a happy feeling of life and mind If you let yourself to forget your own unhappiness, by trying to create a little happiness for others. You are best to yourself. The perfect way to conquer worry is the Prayer of God. To keep yourself from worrying about criticism, do not even try to get mixed with your enemies, because if you do you will hurt yourself far more than we hurting them. Instead of worrying about ingratitude, let's expect it. Let's remember that the only way to find happiness is not to expect gratitude, but to give for the joy of giving. Let us build a happy life within us….generate peace and a healthy atmosphere around us. This will help us to lead a peaceful happy and prosperous life and we would find ourselves to be happier than before. You should do things in the order of their importance. ou need to clear your desk of all papers except those relating to the immediate problem at hand. When you face a problem, solve it then and there, if you have the facts to make a decision. Make a decision fast and do not linger on. Learn to organize, deputize, and supervise and straight away come to decision.

Simply postponing it would spoil your good thoughts and there is every likelihood your mind may get into negative activities and start thinking in negative manner. Therefore write down a list of things that make you excited, however big, small, likely or unlikely. Then work to make them occur more often. Look for moments of joy and savor them. Recognize your good happening every day.Eat well do plenty of exercise and do not skip meals It is a known fact that Physical exercise is known to stimulate our veins and get to strengthen our minds that lift depression and anxiety so we need to walk, swim, run or whatever we like doing best. Those who create or those who do well on the worst scenario, give themselves worry and stress, tend to be devastated. If we cannot get some sunshine, we can always lighten up our rooms with brighter lights. We can have lunch outside the office. Take frequent walks instead of driving our cars over short distances. No man is indispensable. First of all our circle of friends is always there to give us some moral support.

Spending time and engaging ourselves in worthwhile activities could give us a very enjoyable and satisfying feeling. Nothing feels better than having group support. Good friends are quite important and their company generally lightened up our spirits. To get to know and to find such friends we simply have to be friendly with ourselves, and then the friendships will naturally follow us. We need to understand the power of touch and support and we have not to underestimate it strength and support. Don't we feel so good when someone pats us on our back and gives us some words of encouragement during your most challenging times and difficult times. Just hug or embrace someone someday you will see that you have almost changed his life. Get intimate with him and try to establish close ties with his family and friends. The love and care expressed by you will tremendously boost him and well as your immune system and fury of worry will be diminished for all.In our lives storms may come and go in the form of reversals, but if we have the power and foundation of inner fulfillment and if we deal with it with a very clear practical mind these storms will not kill us or will not disrupt us. There could be numberless reasons for which we keep on worrying.

We may be worried about our health, wealth, loved ones, friends, the happening of yesterday and the follow happenings of tomorrow, the environment or the world politics, but these can be dealt with firm mind and fearless worry if we generate within ourselves the power of enlightenment within ourselves.

HAPPINESS LIES IN POSITIVE LIVING
BE POSITVE THINK POSITIVE LIVE POSITIVE
CHAPTER TWENTY NINE
POSITIVITY IS STATE OF MIND

Positivity is something you cannot earn or buy. If you have spent your life trying to get some happiness or something that will make you happy, odds are that you are wasting a really good life that you don't know you have. You passed up and overlooked a lot of personal happiness. You are probably spending so much time chasing and dreaming of unnecessary thing of what could be of no use to you and that you are forgetting about all the small and big things occurring right now that could make you happy. People and things alone, won't make you happy. Your own efforts not to get worried or depressed make you happy. You know the saying, that "Positivity is a state of mind". And state of mind is what you think do and act in a peaceful manner without being getting worried or depressed.The best thing about happiness is that you get it is free. You don't have to pay or you do not have to open any account to be happy. You don't have to pay monthly rent for it either. You just have to change your perspective, your views on what you are seeing and feeling. Happiness is not something which is quite readymade. It comes from your own actions and deeds. Don't let one cloud darken the whole sky. Angriness and happiness don't mix. You must dig out the angriness in you, and see that the happiness has shown and seeded a place to grow its roots. The ultimate goal of life should be to get happiness and not get involved into unnecessary worries falling in the death trap of defeats and failures. The essence of life is not in the great victories and grand failures, but in the simple joys. The purpose of our lives is to be happy. Laugh when you can, apologize when you should, and let go of what you can't change. Think positive and just visualize that what is stored in destiny would not be negative. If you want to be happy, be positive first practice meditation. If you want, others to be happy practice compassion. Whoever is happy will make others happy, too.Let us be very sure and let us keep in mind that happiness doesn't depend on any superficial conditions, it is governed by our mental attitude only. Our greatest gift to others is to be happy and to radiate our happiness to the entire world. Happiness is a guide to direction, not a place to hide. As a happy person, you radiate happiness to the world. Visualize your light radiating throughout the world, passing from person to person until it encircles the globe. Resolve to keep happy, and your joy and you shall form an invincible host against difficulties. The positive persons often dance to the happy tunes of their lives. The path to happiness is forgiveness of everyone and gratitude for everything. Happiness fills your heart each day and your whole life through with clean thoughts. Any day would be a wonderful day if you do not to take life so seriously. Happiness is not about being a winner -it's about being gentle with life being gentle within you. Happiness blooms in the presence of self-respect and the absence of ego. Love yourself. Love everyone around you. Love everyone in the whole world. When you're feeling depressed or anxious, close your eyes and try to visualize a guided positive imaginary thing. First breathe deeply and relax. How important it is to consistently reach for positive, uplifting, inspirational thoughts. Thought that promote aliveness and abundance. Thoughts that make you feel good. Look at the birds of the air; they do not sow or reap or store away in barns, and yet our heavenly Father feeds them. Imagine that you're already a positive person and you love life. The only thing between us and our desire, to be happy, is one single fact: we are not happy because we often fall into the death trap of depression and wholly because of our negative thoughts. Absence of positive thinking, has eluded us of our great happiness and left us far behind. This very little known fact has kept many of us from reaching our goal of happiness. If you keep thinking things like as if your life is dead!", nothing would be achieved and it will be like that only.Throw away all your negative thoughts and worries, concentrate on the goals to be achieved, on the ray of happiness in you and make sure that you are not falling again into the path of negativity. "Happiness is a state of mind only and not the thoughts of negatives, and it quite true that happiness can only be achieved if you have a positive mind and a clear attitude of being a positive person. Happiness and positivity go hand in hand. If you are positive you are a happy person and if you possess negativity you would land yourself to be a very negative person thus ruining your life for what of nothing.

HAPPINESS LIES IN POSITIVE LIVING
BE POSITVE THINK POSITIVE LIVE POSITIVE
CHAPTER THIRTY

DISCARD NEGETIVITY AND BE POSTIVE

You may also feel that life has become terrible for you to live and you are carrying no hope that someone would be there to rescue you. Happiness is your own choice and decision. Each of us can be as happy as we make up our minds to be. We can, if we want, fill up our days with positive attitude chatter and laughter. To be happy, we need to concentrate only on happy thoughts. The ghosts of the past have to be exorcised. You may be working in any field, the key to success is your outlook. Sometimes you may think that no road is left for you from where you can achieve the happiness of life. There may be chances that someone who was there with you before might hold on to you when you are on the dark side of the life. The experience has taught us that we should buy some strength, hope and positive ness from our loved ones to help ourselves in such a situation rather than surrendering as life is a precious gift of God and is equipped with full of joy and happiness if we help ourselves in these critical moments and live with considerable optimism. Happiness in life comes through the doors of positive thoughts; we do not even realize which one is left open. We have so many reasons to cry and at the same time plenty of reasons to smile as well. Keeping our dreams and hope alive might be a reason that success and happiness will come our way again. We ought to know that happiness alone does not stand for anything, but it is on our way of thinking that how do we keep ourselves happy in life. Ending up our lives does not lead us to our destination but of course proves we are supposed to be cowards who know not to unfold the doors of belief in God and in ourselves. Failure and disappointment are part of our life. The only thing is that we need to face and solve the problem. We must not forget to believe in God whatever our situation may be, we would be taken away from Him by the difficulties, in order that we bow down and surrender. But if our faith is strong enough we will not be let down, rather we would break the knees of sorrows and force it to die and lead happy lives. We should not surrender but must find out ways to come out of our worries, anxieties and difficulties. We ought not to indulge ourselves into the darkness of the room but find out the doors to free ourselves from unnecessary fear and worries. We must belief in ourselves and our hearts, and believe in the ones who love us and not the ones whom we love. We must not fall on the negative side of a thing. It is the real time when you keep on revealing the truth of our lives and relations, do not fall on the reverse side but think how good it was that because of the hard times of our lives we could well judge about them. We should always try to be positive and should think that whatever is happening, it is the positive side or consequence of that incident in would be on the positive side of our imagination. With all these thoughts, I would request my readers to implement some good thoughts in their life that would make things easier to be tackled by them. We should accept the situation and fight it with more determination. In this world nothing is good or bad and only thinking makes it so. We ought to know that advice from people around us will help us to overcome from the any drastic situation. Also we have to always minimize the stress as it gives nothing but takes away joy and happiness from our lives. And finally we need to take things casually and fight with it seriously. The next morning after all, will surely come with fresh air to breathe the new hopes in us with the brightness of the sun. A clear minded person looks for good qualities in the other person, whereas a negative mind always looks for the fault in the other person, whereas a negative mind always looks for the fault. An optimist goes forward keeping in mind the past, a pessimist thinks of the future and reverts back to the past. In fact negative thoughts are our greatest enemies. Experience the happiness in all circumstances by maintaining better relationships. How about understanding that sadness cannot touch a person with a positive attitude? The capability increases as It boosts up patience and confidence. It increases the decision of making power. Creative way of thoughts appears in the mind. Positive thoughts teach the art of finding solutions to any problem. Optimism is something what we do. Anxiety and other negative emotions are known to be detrimental to the body, especially to our immune systems, and having an optimistic nature seems to protect against those effects. People who are supposed to be optimistic, about their future, behaving differently. They do exercise, do not indulge in in smoking and often follow a good and better diet. Whenever we are unhappy, if we analyze the reason for our unhappiness, it is because life is not matching our expectations.

HAPPINESS LIES IN POSITIVE LIVING
BE POSITVE THINK POSITIVE LIVE POSITIVE
CHAPTER THIRTY ONE
STOP WORRYING BE POSITIVE

Is it true that do you constantly worry about what people think of you?. If yes, then you need to follow these tips to get over your worries: We need to know and realize that nobody is perfect or flawless. If we try to change the way we look, talk and behave just to please others, and show our pride we will gradually become such a person that we ourselves won't recognize each other and would start and create unnecessary worries within us and our surrounding without being positive and will not start to live happily. We ought to stop worrying over unnecessary things be positive and live without fear happily. We need to understand that what people think of us is their concern, and not ours. If they think about us to be, too reticent or proud, it's really not our business. If every time we happen to meet some new fellows, we may wonder and imagine as what they think of us, and with this feeling in us we will never be able to live a trouble-free and hassle free life. We are bound to fall into the trap of unnecessary worries denying us the startup of new and the happy living life. We must think rationally. Is it in our hands or can we control what others think about us?. Simply we need to ignore them If we cannot, and live our lives the way we want to and find the ways to leave worries aside and start living a happy life. Let us make our way to happy living. It is a well-known fact that attitude decides how a natives or persons copes up with the day to day events of life. Attitude is what a influence a person's reaction to a situation in life is. It sets the emotional undertone for a person to his likes or dislikes a situation even before he is acquainted with it. Positive attitude is a quality that is second to none in a human being. We acknowledge our children to say a big thank you from the time to time irrespective they being very little, we teach them to be grateful for everything that they receive. We attach so much importance to this attitude of gratitude that when our children fail to thank someone, we insist that they do it. That is what is needed to be avoided from time to time. We expect this in return from others when we help them or give them a gift. We call a person discourteous and rude when they do not say thank us in return. Though we attach so much importance to this attitude, as we grow into teenage and adult years we find ourselves becoming ungrateful or taking things for granted. We lose touch with the very same qualities that we instill in our children. We take for granted our life, our health, our families, the people in our lives, the things that our loved ones do for us to make our lives easier and things that we possess. The attitude of positive speaks a lot about a person. It denotes about changing negative attitudes and making positive thinking a positive attitude a good habit. Thinking positively and a positive attitude help us to appreciate and value ourselves, our potential and all that we have. It ensures that we do not take our abilities for granted. It makes us look at ourselves as special people with a special set of abilities and potential. It banishes the feelings of inadequacy and insecurity that arises from unfair comparisons with others. It helps us to appreciate people for who they are and not magnify what they are not and their little flaws. It drives away prejudice and makes us approach life with an open mind. It predisposes us to react to the daily events of life in a positive manner and help us to look at the brighter side of life. Make us optimistic. It gives hope and helps us look forward to life with anticipation.

We need to know that positive thinking takes the focus away from what we don't have, to appreciating and making good use of what we have. It is closely connected to our emotional wellbeing and happiness. We feel loved and at peace with ourselves for a major part of our lives when we make this attitude ours. This adds and helps us to get rid of greed, amenity, bitterness, jealousy, and promotes a healthy and nurturing attitude towards others, which in turn gets reciprocated and we feel the sense of healthy living. On the face of it we ought to know that a positive is not an attitude of being satisfied and content, that you never want to do anything, anymore. This is an attitude that makes you feel good about who you are, what you do, and what your potentials are. This attitude impels you to utilize all that you are endowed with as a person, to achieve the highest possible goals. When we have this attitude, we are able to work without any external pressure to perform but there is sufficient pressure and motivation from within. The possessing of positive thinking is like any other habit, so we need to follow the routine of habit formation here as well. You will win new friends and admirers without having to impress them or conform to the pressure of doing things their way. You will be bubbling with life and the joie de vivre. You will be rearing to go and accomplish all you can with your new found confidence. The best part of adopting the 'positive thinking and a positive attitude of gratitude is that, you will be able to enjoy the smallest pleasures of nature with a heightened sense of satisfaction and awe. I can see and watch a beautiful flower and carry that joy in my mind for future enjoyment with a clear positive habit. I can go back to work freshen and can use it as an object to meditate on when I feel stressed.Let us be clear that a positive is not an attitude of being satisfied and content, that you never want to do anything, anymore. This is an attitude that makes you feel good about who you are, what you do, and what your potentials are. This attitude impels you to utilize all that you are endowed with as a person, to achieve the highest possible goals. When we have this attitude, we are able to work without any external pressure to perform but there is sufficient pressure and motivation from within. The habit of positive thinking is like any other habit, so we need to follow the routine of habit formation here as well.

HAPPINESS LIES IN POSITIVE LIVING

BE POSITVE THINK POSITIVE LIVE POSITIVE

CHAPTER THIRTY TWO

WHY DISAPPOINTMENT

Why Disappointment and Negative Thinking

At time we may think that there is no road is left for us from where we can achieve the happiness of our lives. We may also feel that life has become terrible for us to live and we are carrying new hope that someone would come to rescue us. There may be chances that someone who was there with us before might have held on to us when we were on the dark side of the life. We should not forget that happiness in life comes through the doors of positive thoughts; we need to have them first. If one door happen to close, another opens, in the event only when we are confident and optimistic. We have so many reasons to cry and at the same time plenty of reasons to smile as well. Similarly, happiness does not stand for anything, but is on our way of thinking that how do we keep ourselves happy in life. Failure and disappointment are part of our life. The only thing is that we need to face and solve the problem is by keeping our dreams and hope alive be it a reason that success and happiness will come our way again.The experience has taught us that we should buy some strength, hope and positivity from our loved ones to help ourselves in such a situation rather than surrendering as life is a precious gift of God and is equipped with full of joy and happiness if we help ourselves in these critical moments we can live with considerable optimism. What if when everything goes wrong and all the doors of happiness are closed our live becomes a silent. It is a quite common and we are aware of a marvelous proverb that Life itself is a stage and we all are the performers, performing different acts assigned to us by our almighty power. We should not forget as to what is in our possession?, if it is to fulfill our duties towards our responsibility and do whatever is correct and is allowed by us in our life?. However, despite of all these good thoughts which are embodied to us by the almighty fail to revive these unwanted circumstances that lead us to sorrow and difficulties and a situation where we do not know what is correct and good for us and what is wrong for us. We should always remember that, "Life is there, where there is hope". That single thing that remains in our hands is to find out ways to know how to overcome these worries of our life at that very moment when all doors are closed for us which means that whatever situation is there, we must not give up hope. We must fight because there have been always a chance that with good faith and hard work we can turn the odds in our favor. It is often said that it is very easy to advise but when it comes to us, things go out of our control and we fail to suggest a way out for ourselves. We fall into the trap of unnecessary worries and elope ourselves with negative thoughts. We feel better when somebody else is facing some difficulty but when it comes to us we fail to gather that faith, will power and the words of strength. It is a common fact that no one in this world is free of obstacles or difficulties. If all the openings of happiness are shut for us and we have to overcome that and have no way to come out, but to survive lest we must have to learn to swim out of the sorrows because this is what is called life and sorrow free living. There are lot more examples and in many other situations, where we will find that how we could have faced and fought with our sorrows and difficulties of life when there was no hope left in our lives. When the power of will is at the worst and each one of us knows that the one who is gone never comes back. Neither a thousands of words would not be enough to bring him back nor a million tears, because each and every moment, eyes would only shed tears , mind would remain tensed and we would be simply surrounded by worries and the life seems to have been vanished. Life is ever expanding, contraction is death. As commonly said by big saints that the self- seeking man who is looking after his personal comforts and leading a lazy life for himself there would be no room for him even in the hell and he simply have lost the power of his will.

We are quite aware of the fact that faith in oneself is the history of a man and that faith calls the quality of superiority within a person. One cannot do anything without it. We fail only when we do not try very hard to achieve the power and faith within us. As soon as we lose faith, death comes in our way and we are surrounds by all the evils and stupid worries of the world.The secret and history of every successful man is to have, good confidence, faith and strength behind him and that remain the right cause of his single success in life. Unselfishness plays a very vital role in his life. He may not have been perfectly unselfish, yet he was tending towards it. If he had been perfectly unselfish, he would have been as great a success. The degree of unselfishness marks the degree of success everywhere and he leads to be successful man without fear worries and selfishness. There are quite a number of reasons to believe that for a successful and happy life the mystery surrounding it lies in our interests, and good memory which is the basis of our interest, power of desire and aim, keeping ourselves smiling and the doubt free character which is the foremost important reason for a successful and happy life. If we possess one solid unselfish and doubt free character within ourselves we would be quite happy and successful. The love for God and worshipping God adds to one common thing the immense faith in Him. There may be different beliefs and ways to worship God in different communities, places and religions, but one thing remains the same and that is the Love of God for all of us. Our world is full of odds and evens, happiness and sorrows, fulfilment and emptiness. And these are all created by the Almighty. However, the most beautiful Gift of God, is Human, which is such a mystery driven by Him which could hardly be defined or explained in depth. We know that life cannot be foreseen. Life is not a bed of roses. Life is a battle field and not a bed of roses as every man on earth has to struggle very hard in making his life happy. If aim of our life is to stay happy and let others to be happy, we will be happy and remembered by all. But no one will actually remember us for the wealth we have gained, or success we have achieved. I have no aim in life. Summary living with no purpose in life is just like a feather moving towards the wind. Both career and purpose are different issues but it is equally important to understand the value of these things which would ultimately add spicy flavor to your living. Innovation at work place is what is it necessary how well we judge our work, how good we like and enjoy it. If we take our work as a stiff challenge and as learning everyday then we would start loving it and giving our best. However, if we just work for the sake of then nothing is realized and we do not remain happy in life.Life is such a special gift of Almighty and it is not gifted by Him to use it the way we like or love to. The actual path shown by Him needs to be followed by us for us to reach the peak of betterment every moment. We need to have some positive attitude to look at it comfortably but at the same time having a positive mental attitude does not mean banishing all negative thoughts and people from your life. The same is true with thoughts. When we go to field with negative thoughts, we banish one and another one arises. Therefore creation of positivity in life is utmost necessary to enjoy the special gift of God to us.Now let's us imagine that we are not feeling at our best today, and we are having thoughts that could be classified as negative. We shouldn't be thinking such negative thoughts. We don't like the negative thoughts. We ought to know that negative thoughts are stressful, demoralizing and depressing. We shouldn't aim to have negative thoughts at all. Often we feel uncomfortable because we think we have to say or do something in response to another person's words. When we find ourselves thinking this way, it helps enormously to take a few moments to check inside and notice what we are feeling. We are deeply depressed that negativity has governed us and has taken a deep root in our minds.....

HAPPINESS LIES IN POSITIVE LIVING
BE POSITVE THINK POSITIVE LIVE POSITIVE
CHAPTER THIRTY THREE
STEPS FOR HAPPY LIFE AND POSITIVITY

The secret of successful and happy life lies in keeping ourselves smiling and the character which is the foremost important reason that lies within us. Do not be curious about anything, but in everything, by prayer and petition, with thanksgiving, present your requests to God. Whenever your mind is tempted to jump the fence and start to worry, say this verse aloud or to yourself. You may even have to repeat it over and over again. Am I constantly striving to see the positive in every aspect of my life?. Steps for a successful and happy life. We need to believe that a Positive Attitude is a choice. This step is hard to take. People are either positive or negative. They tend to blame their negativity on all kinds of outside forces—fate, experiences, parents, relationship, but never really stopped to think that they could choose to be positive. Piercing ourselves that positivity is a choice has been one of the greatest things we have ever done for ourselves. Now when we find ourselves in a bad situation, we know that it's up to us to find the good, to be positive regardless of what's happening around us. We should no longer point fingers and place blame to anyone else. We need to realize that everything happens how it happens, and it's up to us to choose how we want to feel about it. We need to be in control of our attitude, and no one can take that away this from us.If we want to live a positive, joyful life, we must not be surrounded by negative people who don't encourage our happiness. As a negative person, we ought to get attracted too negative people only. Only when we decide to make the change to live a more positive life, we have to get rid of our lives of the most negative influences in it. We are quite aware of the fact that no one is perfect and perfection isn't the goal when it comes to positivity but there were people in our lives who were consistently negative, who constantly bring us down, we need to stop spending so much time with them. We can very well imagine, it is not easy for us to get away from these negative people. It can hurt us to keep distance from people even when you know they aren't good for us and for our current lifestyle. In addition to removing negative influences from them, we also have to get rid of some of our own negative behaviors, such as the drug and alcohol abuse. We need to take some concrete steps and examine which behaviors are good for us and which were not harmful. What we need is to learn to focus on the positive things, such as working on positive activities and cultivating new, positive relationships. We must let go of the negative ones. This process may be not easy to live a positive life when negative people and behaviors continually pull us down.In every situation or in every person there is something good. Most of the time it's not easy to find the positive qualities but we have to look hard to discover positivity in them. Now, when we are faced with a difficult or challenging situation, we need to think and talk to ourselves and console our mind, no matter how terrible the situation might seem, we can always find something good if we take the time to think about it. It is quite obvious that anything good and bad is learning experience so, at the very least, we must learn from bad experiences. However, there's usually even more to it than that. If you really take some time to have a look at it, we would find something good, something genuinely positive, about every person or situation. Once we start thinking more positively, we will realize that we had to reinforce these thoughts and behaviors within ourselves so that we could stick to it. As with any sort of training, the more we practice, the better we get to be positive. The best and easiest way to do this is to be positive when it comes to who we are. We need to speak to ourselves that we are awesome. And we have done a good job at work thus creating positivity within us. We need to be honest with ourselves, and we need to do our best to look for the good. And, whatever we do, we must not focus on the negative. It is alright not to like everything about ourselves, but don't focus on what we don't like. We have all the positive attributes, and it's up to us to remind ourselves of them every day.

Not only do we need to be positive with ourselves for this multiple action to take effect, but we need to be more positive with others. We have to share our wealth of positivity with the people of the world. The best way is to be nice with other people, no matter what. Tell them that they look nice today. Appreciate their job and tell them that have done a great job on that assignment. Be positive and tell your elder or your kids how much you love them and how great they are. When someone is feeling down, do what we need to do is to cheer him or her up. Do send them gifts nice flower and glow them with nice notes. What is required is that we never wanted to see the good in ourselves and, therefore, didn't want to see it in others also. We must not be critical and condescending rather we must be encouraging and supportive. We should not try to treat others as we would like to be treated, but also try to consider how we would like to be treated. The world likes to appreciate positivity, and the more we share it with others, the more we would be practicing it your own lives. When we start feeling like the idea of not being a positive person we need to remind ourselves that all it takes is one tiny step in the right direction to move towards a more positive attitude. We have to believe in ourselves and remember the most important lesson of all is a positive outlook and that is a choice that we can always make. The power of remaining positive, whatever the situation, can never be underestimated. We are all here for a short duration, but is it worth it to spend any of that time in a any angry or being negative?. That need to sort out in mind and soul and thus must share our positive thoughts with others. The real test of any one is to remain positive whenever some challenges become difficult. Remaining positive keeps our mind in the right state of balance and often opens resolutions to the problems at hand. Negativity is contagious and spreads like fire. It not only does its affect anyone, but it spreads to everyone who ever comes in contact with it or whoever they interact with. When only the negative perspective is in focus, the resolution process is impeded. Eliminating negativity, or rather, being positive is a mindset that can be found at any moment, and which can be turned into a habit. We must throw away the negativity in us and opt for being a very positive person.

HAPPINESS LIES IN POSITIVE LIVING
BE POSITVE THINK POSITIVE LIVE POSITIVE
CHAPTER THIRTY FOUR
MAKE YOUR WAY FROM
NEGATIVITY TO POSTIVITY

We need to learn a lesson from every situation. No matter how difficult the situation may appear. We should recognize the beautiful lessons waiting to be discovered. Sometimes lessons may prove to be expensive and costly, but every problem is a learning experience in disguise. We need to be conscious of our thoughts, especially, when life just isn't going our way. The moment we see that we are diving into frustration, agony, sorrow or low self –esteem we must shift our thoughts, by thinking about something completely different and unrelated. This will strangle the pattern of self-pity, mind-created imaginations, and negative downward stairs. Really what makes us different from other mammals is our ability to control our thoughts and think for ourselves positively and shift our negative thoughts to a positive angle. We may have made mistakes, but now we can accept it and continue, knowing that we will make a different decision in the future. If we understand this it can be appreciative for the experience. We cannot be both angry and grateful at the same time. We should start counting the blessings and miracles in our lives and if we start exploring for them and we would find more. We should console our mind as to what's not there to be grateful?. It's quite true that we are alive and breathing! We have to realize how lucky we are with all the positivity in abundance in our lives. Our mind and body becomes dumb and mum when it comes to pressure, all it wants to do is take the easiest way out and to throw out of us our negative within us. Feeling good about ourselves and showing self-confidence boosts our skills potential and capabilities in any areas of work and supports us to become more positive. We need to shift our thoughts from being a negative person to more strong a positive man. Also keeping in mind that pushing things to the limit and going beyond what we think is possible for us to get to the next step of being positive. It becomes another key to achieving what we really want to do. Even if it may even be relationships and we are finding it difficult to meet someone where we are actually interested in, we need not wait because it usually doesn't come to us by own, we must stand up to get help from any learned fellow. One of the most important things while doing all of this is to be happy about what we are doing, thus we ought to have a successful goal setting our lifestyle with a positive attitude. At times we may suffer from chronic depression, though we know how good things look on to others life cannot be worse for us. Let's imagine how to deal when life leaves a great big steaming pile at our doorstep. Lest we need to remember that external factors can be dealt with by taking positive steps to repair or at least address the root of the problem as best as we can. Whatever may be the primary cause of the problem, that cause must be examined first?. We may or may not be able to solve the problem, per se, but at least knowing that we are taking positive steps can help us improve our outlook. It will not be easy, of course, for us and it may be like suffering a chronic disease thus we must balance ourselves as "being positive" with an understanding that the reality is, it's going to be an ongoing battle for our own survival. Depression will undermine even the strongest of wills, need help to maintain or at least be reminded of a positive outlook. Counseling, psychotherapy, and the right combination of medication will play a crucial role in helping to keep us from sinking into that very dark place that is the essence of depression. Be patient, but don't look for miracles. It may be that we will need the help of professionals throughout our lives to maintain a generally even keel. If one could "will away" depression, there would be no need of doctors or drugs. What we can do is understand why we feel like we do, and explain to our counselors that we wish it were that easy, and that we appreciate our concern towards positivity. Shifting our thoughts enables us to the right path of our positivity and thinking in its direction of positivity can make us to lead a very happy life.

HAPPINESS LIES IN POSITIVE LIVING
BE POSITVE THINK POSITIVE LIVE POSITIVE
CHAPTER THIRTY FIVE

EAT WELL AND BE HAPPY

We need to remember that as we possibly as we can we should make it a point to eat a more balanced, and healthy diet even though we may very little money left with us. We have intake of lot of greens vegetables and with variety of fruit and nuts which are all super healthy food for us, and which are less expensive than meats, cheeses, and processed foods! Their nitrifying value will energize and elevate our body, and knowing this that we are treating ourselves will surely refresh our minds. If we look for rich food rich in vitamins and other useful ingredients which include nuts, soya beans and fatty fish we would get more nutrition value. We must cut back on the caffeine drinks, alcohol. We don't have to quit, but reducing the intake of them will help reduce anxiety and stress from time to time.Exercise is one of health sport that our body needs most. It may be yoga, cross training, or even a simple walking in the park. This helps keeping our body active and will also help to grow our outlook. If we make it hobby we would enjoy the most. Whether its art, photography, music focusing on something other than the worry factor it will give our mind some good atmosphere to breathe off and would generate a good behavior within us. The other refreshing factor is naturally our sleep. We need not be reminded of this. Our body is probably begging us for it when we are in the middle of hard times. We may be drawn to maintain good sleeping habits. Maintain a consistent sleep schedule, but allow yourself some leeway. If we sleep peacefully let our body get about 8 hours of sleep we get the best results. If you're just starting to have those thoughts, speak to your physician or your therapist. They may prescribe something to help steer you back to the center, emotionally. It may be the act of talking about it is therapeutic enough, but don't assume that. Leave that call to the professionals. Having goals which are set again and again after each one is achieved will give you a mindset or target to strive for which leads to success, with success becomes natural positive attitude. With all costiveness, goals and success builds a higher potential and belief within yourself. Setting realistic goals that you know you can achieve by staying positive is a great beginning to success. Your attitude around your friends, family and public people really tells them who you are, being positive instead of negative makes an excellent first impression on anybody. Positive means to be absolute, clear-cut, definite, forward-looking and expressively firm with a decision. Having a positive attitude toward something means you are willing to commit and do the work without complaint, which leads to goals. You realize that what appears negative today will change tomorrow. Nothing stays the same. Whether you are positive or negative, the situation does not change. So, we mind as well be positive. As with any habit, the habit of remaining positive in all situations takes practice and a commitment to yourself to take control. But start small, start paying attention to your emotions, start by wanting to change. Communicate each other with positive talksIf you have a problem, the thing to do is to communicate: find out the information you need to get the full picture, so that the solution becomes apparent. If you're upset, you need to communicate and say how you feel. If you've done something wrong, again you need to communicate The nature of this world is that we have to face birth, old age, disease and death. Everything is always changing. The biggest problem is that we want to control our environment. Don't hold onto anything that bothers your mind. It can only hurt your health and it won't help your problems at all. The people that live the longest in this world do not hold grudges or hold onto negative feelings. Visualize your worries on a large chalkboard in your mind. Watch yourself take a big eraser and erase the problems. Every time the thoughts come back into your head, see yourself with the eraser again. Keep your slate clean! "Worry does not empty tomorrow of its sorrow, it empties today of its strength. ""If a problem is fixable, if a situation is such that you can do something about it, then there is no need to worry. If it's not fixable, then there is no help in worrying. There is no benefit in worrying whatsoever. Worrying is carrying tomorrow's load with today's strength- carrying two days at once. It is moving into tomorrow ahead of time. Worrying doesn't empty tomorrow of its sorrow, it empties today of its strength." "If we are worried about the future, then we must look today at the upbringing of children. "Life is what you make it, so make it a happy one!! Don't worry on things that may not happen, life is too short to worry too much. Smile and be happy recent studies have shown that smiling cause's natural body chemicals to increase that can increase your good health. You receive the same benefits whether you feel like smiling or not. Smiling also benefits everyone that sees it. Smiling at others makes them feel good too. So smile, fake or not, it is good for you and good for your recipient. It is the best medicine. Based on the same concept above about smiling, laughing burns calories, increases your adrenaline and boosts health. There are even groups of people that get together just to laugh together. They are not laughing at jokes, they are just laughing for good health. As with smiling, you do not need to laugh at real things, you just need to do the physical laughing for all of the health benefits. Even small amounts of exercise make you feel better. Take a walk if you are feeling bluesy, angry or think you may be slipping into negative thinking. Getting your blood pumping empowers you to do what you need to do and to do what's right. Set a schedule of regular exercise at least 3 days a week for at least 20 minutes each session for better health. See articles below for starting a fitness program. Even a little bit helps, if you need to start out small, that is fine, just walk for 10 minutes a day and slowly increase it.

HAPPINESS LIES IN POSITIVE LIVING

BE POSITVE THINK POSITIVE LIVE POSITIVE

CHAPTER THIRTY SIX

ROLL BACK YOUR HAPPY DAYS

FORGET NEGATIVITY

BE POSITIVE

Don't hold onto anything that bothers your mind. It can only hurt your health and it won't help your problems at all. The people that live the longest in this world do not hold grudges or hold onto negative feelings. Visualize your worries on a large chalkboard in your mind. Watch yourself take a big eraser and erase the problems. Every time the thoughts come back into your head, see yourself with the eraser again. Keep your slate clean! Therefore do not worry about tomorrow, for tomorrow will worry about itself. Each day has enough trouble of its own. Do not anticipate trouble, or worry about what may never happen. Keep in the sunlight. Imagine every day to be the last of a life surrounded with hopes, cares, anger and fear. The hours that come unexpectedly will be much the more grateful.The mind that is anxious about future events is miserable. Present fears are less than horrible imaginings. Let us be of good cheer, remembering that the misfortunes hardest to bear are those that never happen, focus on the positive aspects of their lives, rather than on the negative setbacks. "Feeling confident affects the way we perceive our situations and how we decide to manage them. Don't waste your life in doubts and fears: spend yourself on the work before you, well assured that the right performance of this hour's duties will be the best preparation for the hours or ages that follow it.It is not work that kills men, it is worry. Work is healthy; you can hardly put more on a man than he can bear. But worry is rust upon the blade. It is not movement that destroys the machinery, but friction.Never let life's hardships disturb you ... no one can avoid problems, not even saints or sages. As with any habit, the habit of remaining positive in all situations takes practice and a commitment to yourself to take control.Life is what you make it, so make it a happy one!! Don't worry on things that may not happen, life is to short to worry to much. Smile and be happy

HAPPINESS LIES IN POSITIVE LIVING
BE POSITVE THINK POSITIVE LIVE POSITIVE
CHAPTER THIRTY SEVEN
WHAT IS WORRY?

Thought which are provoking our mind, about the uncertainties and the negativities, as to what will happen tomorrow. Worries are repetitive thoughts associated with feelings of anxiety in anticipation of some negative future event. Whether the worries are about financial crisis, family problems, work, health or any topic of concern, the anxious feelings produced and sustained by the imaginary thoughts which always distinctly appear to be unpleasant. Worrying will carry tomorrow's load with today's strength. Worry will not empty tomorrow of its sorrows, it empties today of its power and strength. Worries make you to move into tomorrow ahead of time. Half the worry in the world is caused by people trying to make decisions before they have sufficient knowledge on which to base a decision. Why worry about the future. Just imagine as to what if we just acted like everything was easy and there was nothing very serious about it to come in future. Worry often gives a small thing a big shadow and its surrounding do frightened with more scary things. Why worry about tomorrow; concentrate on today happening as for tomorrow will worry about itself. Each day has its own worries and troubles. If there is not any solution to the some problem then do not waste time worrying about it. And if there is a solution to the problem then why waste time worrying about it. Worry will never rob tomorrow of its sorrows, but will only deny today of its meaning happiness and joys. Worrying is actually a form of superstition and creates false images in our mind and that is the main reason and cause which makes and leads us to this point of imagination. A human being can survive almost anything, as long as he or she sees the end in sight. If something bad or good is to happen it is sure to happen, whether we worry or not. Let us put our energy into today and stop worrying about the future and past. We should not foresee trouble, or worry about what may never happen as past is dead and gone forever and future is uncertain and yet to come. The basic facts we should know about worry. The basic techniques to analyze worry and how to break the worry habit before it breaks us. These are the simple ways where we can concentrate and get rid of worries prevailing in our thoughts. Annalise worry to see and get the reasons and facts of worry. To avoid reoccurrence of worries, concentrate on prayers as prayers are the best source of remedies of the prevailing worries. The more you pray, the less you'll panic. The more you worship, the less you worry. There is nothing that wastes the body like worry, and anyone who has any faith in God should need not to worry about anything whatsoever is to happen in future. We ought to know the basic fundamental of analyzing worries. Worries create unnecessary thoughts and these are caused by people going in for unwanted decisions, fore hand not even knowing as to when a good decision is made and not even having sufficient knowledge about it. We must first study and after carefully weighing all the facts than only come to a powerful decision. Simply making castles in the air won't solve our problems but add more to our vows. Anxiety and worry can go hand in hand.

When anxiety grabs the mind, it is self-perpetuating. Your mind gets clogged with numerous with buts and ifs. Do not worry about your life. Worries are repetitive thoughts associated with feelings of anxiety in anticipation of some negative future event.

Yet anxious feelings and the worries that lead to them can prove helpful. It becomes a difficult problem if you are constantly anxious as it will become a hindrance to your everyday life, rather than motivate you to some good and better things. Never worry alone. Worrisome thoughts reproduce faster so one of the most powerful ways to stop the spiral of worry is simply to disclose the worry to a friend. What you will eat or drink; or about your body, what you will wear. If you know that the circumstance is beyond your control or power change than revise it to your liking. Just try to put a stop-less order on your worries. Don't permit little things which become insects of life to ruin your happiness. Co-operate with the inevitable. Decide just how much anxiety a thing may be worth and refuse to give in anymore. All the happiness is not given in one go it comes slowly and slowly. If your worries center on, an important relationship in your life, pay special attention to remain positive and be happy. To keep yourself happy, treat your worried thoughts as valuable signals. How to keep from worrying about criticism? Simply unjust criticism is often a disguised compliment.

It often means that you have aroused jealousy and envy. Let's keep a record of the fool things we have done and criticize ourselves. The utmost cause of worry is your state of depression. Worries are there to motivate information-gathering and problem-solving. Depression is the inability to construct a future. Depression is inertia. That's the thing about depression: But depression is so insidious, and it compounds daily, that it's impossible to ever see the end. Depressed people think they know themselves, but maybe they only know depression. There are no hopeless than this to get depressed. Our attitude towards suffering and depression becomes very important because it can affect how we cope with suffering when it arises. Depression is nourished by a lifetime of un grieved and unforgiven causes. Never worry about your heart till it stops beating. How can you deal with anxiety? You might try what when you did. A person worried so much that he decided to hire someone to do his worrying for him. Times will change for the better when you change. Worry is a misuse of the imagination. Worry is most often a prideful way of thinking that you have more control over life and its circumstances than you actually do. To keep yourself happy, treat your worried thoughts as valuable signals. These are the fundamental facts you should be familiar about worries. A huge factor to stay happy is to cater your worries around, an important relationship in your life and pay special attention sustaining positive relationships. Worries are there to motivate information gathering and problem-solving. Make your mind firm and do come to a positive decision as come what we will not allow the worries to entire our mind and soul. Once a decision is carefully reached we should get busy carrying out our decisions and should not bother about all the anxieties that are about to come. When we, or any of our colleagues or associates, are about to worry about a problem, we must write it out and think of the following questions: Instead of worrying about what people say of you, why not spend time trying to accomplish something they will admire. What if we just acted like everything was easy? How would your life be different if you stopped worrying about things we can't control and started focusing on the things we can? Let today be the day. You free yourself from fruitless worry, seize the day and take effective action on things you can change…

HAPPINESS LIES IN POSITIVE LIVING

BE POSITVE THINK POSITIVE LIVE POSITIVE

CHAPTER THIRTY EIGHT

WHAT DO YOU GET OUT OF WORRYING?

You may feel largely uncomfortable, when worries attack your thoughts and mind which makes worrying about a situation an easier option to get depressed and diffused. While you are consuming more worries you are far too busy to do anything else to fix the real problem and would rather find it hard to get into a smart solution. Thus resulting in a fact that you spend your evenings worrying only without even bothering to find some time to search a new job. You get nothing out of worrying except only to think and cry. Another cause of getting worried is the attachment with which your inner soul gets attracted to. Attachment brings worry. If you have a problem and you come up with the answer, you stop worrying immediately. Our minds can be dishonest, persuading us that we are worrying about something, when our deepest fear is entirely different. No-one likes to admit that they've chosen to worry. The first step is to write down your worries, which will help you make sense of them, and then decide on one small step you can take towards a solution. But to be very true no man in this world is free of obstacles or difficulties. Don't make worry your habit. Break this habit and stop all the negative and panic thoughts provoking your mind all the time. If you can't change the past, but you must not ruin the present by worrying about the future. Joy is what happens to us when we allow ourselves to recognize how good things really are. When we feel worried and depressed, we need to consciously form a smile on our faces and act upbeat until the

happy feeling becomes genuine reality. Feelings of depression and hopelessness and or anger are even tougher to cope with on a consistent basis. When you are worried, you not only hurt yourself, but the limited support systems that are still holding on your mind but making you to get more and more worried and nothing is achieved in terms of success except the re-carnation of worries and worries. Your actions breed confidence and courage. If you want to conquer fear, anger and worry do not sit ideal and just think about it. Let our deep worrying become advance thinking and planning. If you look into your own mind and heart, and you find nothing wrong there, what is there to worry about? Practically nothing what is there to fear about and again nothing? So why worry unnecessarily and make your present and future dark.

HAPPINESS LIES IN POSITIVE LIVING

BE POSITVE THINK POSITIVE LIVE POSITIVE

CHAPTER THIRTY NINE

WHY WORRY SO MUCH

Negative thought which are provoking our mind, about the uncertainties and the negativities, as to what will happen tomorrow creates unnecessary worries and worries are repetitive thoughts associated with feelings of anxiety in anticipation of some negative future event which may end in a failure. Whether the worries are about financial crisis, family problems, work, health or any topic of concern, the anxious feelings and negative thoughts produced are always distinctly unpleasant. Annalise positive thinking and stop worry over petty matters. Worrying will carry tomorrow's load with today's strength. Worry will not empty tomorrow of its sorrows, but it tends to empty today of its power and strength. Worries make you to move into tomorrow ahead of time. Half the worry in the world is caused by people trying to make decisions before they have sufficient knowledge on which to base a decision. Their negative thoughts pressurize them to be away from the positivity in their lives as they fail and do not analysis on positive

Generate Positive Thinking

Why worry about the future. Just imagine as to what if we just acted like everything was easy and there was nothing very serious about it to come in future. Worry often gives a small thing a big shadow and its surrounding do frightened with more scary things. Why worry about tomorrow; concentrate on today happening as for tomorrow will worry about itself. Each day has its own worries and troubles. Always think positive. If there is not any solution to the some problem then do not waste time worrying about it. And if there is a solution to the problem then why waste time worrying about it. Act fast be positive generate positive thinking worries will automatically vanish in the air. But if you tend to worry they will never rob tomorrow of its sorrows, but will only deny today of its meaning happiness and joys. Negative thoughts only produce worries and worrying is actually a form of superstition and creates false images in our mind and that is the main reason and cause which makes and leads us to this point of imagination. A human being can survive almost anything, as long as he or she sees the end in sight and starts analyzing his positive thoughts. We must not forgot that ff something bad or good is to happen it is sure to happen, whether we worry or not. Let us put our energy into today and stop worrying about the future and past. We should not foresee trouble, or worry about what may never happen as past is dead and gone forever and future is uncertain and yet to come. Positive Thinking will ward off everything and bring happiness in our lives. The basic facts we should know about worry. The basic techniques to analyze worry and how to break the worry habit before it breaks us. These are the simple ways where we can concentrate and get rid of worries prevailing in our thoughts.

Think Positive and Pray- Why Worry?

Annalise positive thinking by annualizing worry you get to see and get the reasons and facts of worry. To avoid reoccurrence of worries, concentrate on prayers as prayers are the best source of remedies of the prevailing worries. Think Positive and Pray. The more you pray, the less you'll panic. The more you worship, the less you worry. There is nothing that wastes the body like worry, and anyone who has any faith in God should need not to worry about anything whatsoever is to happen in future. Positive thinking is the creation of good imagination. We must first study and after carefully weighing all the facts than only come to a powerful decision. Simply making castles in the air won't solve our problems but add more to our vows. Anxiety and worry can go hand in hand. When anxiety grabs the mind, it is self-perpetuating. Your mind gets clogged with numerous with buts and ifs. Do not worry about your life. Worries are repetitive thoughts associated with feelings of anxiety in anticipation of some negative future event. Yet anxious feelings and the worries that lead to them can prove helpful. It becomes a difficult problem if you are constantly anxious to know as to the happening of the future. It will become a hindrance to your everyday life, rather than motivate you to some good and better things. Worrisome thoughts reproduce faster so one of the most powerful ways to stop the spiral of worry is simply to disclose the worry to a friend. What you eat or drink; or about your body, what you will wear will add to negativity may discard positive thinking.

Happiness comes with Positive Thinking.

If you know that the circumstance is beyond your control or power change than revise it to your liking. Just try to put a stop-less order on your worries. Don't permit little things which become insects of life to ruin your happiness. Co-operate with the inevitable. Decide just how much anxiety a thing may be worth and refuse to give in anymore. All the happiness is not given in one go it comes slowly and slowly with positive thinking. Have worry under your control. If your worries center around, pay special attention to remain positive and be happy. Keep yourself happy, treat your worried thoughts as valuable signals. How to keep from worrying about criticism?. Simply unjust criticism and think positively and do often discard a bad compliment. It often means that you have aroused jealousy and envy. Let's keep a record of the fool things we have done and stop criticizing ourselves.

Cause of Worry is Negative Thinking- Think Positive

The utmost cause of worry is our negative thinking as it leads us to the state of depression. Worries are there to motivate us and not a mere source of information-gathering and problems. Dejection and Depression is the inability to construct a future. Depression is inertia. That's the thing about depression: But depression is so insidious, and it compounds daily, that it's impossible to ever see the end. Depressed people think they know themselves, but maybe they only know depression. There are no hopeless than this to get depressed. They never even attempt to think positive.

Times will change for the better-Think Positive

Our negative thinking and attitude towards suffering and depression becomes very important because it can affect how we cope with suffering when it arises. Depression is nourished by a lifetime of un-grieved and unforgiven causes. Never worry about your heart till it stops beating. How can you deal with anxiety? You might try what when you did. A person worried so much that he decided to hire someone to do his worrying for him. Times will change for the better when you change. Worry is a misuse of the imagination. Worry is most often a prideful way of thinking that you have more control over life and its circumstances than you actually do. Positive Thinking leads your way to good and happiness. An art of Good and Happy Living.Neglect worries keep yourself happy, treat your worried thoughts as valuable signals. These are the fundamental facts you should be familiar about worries. A huge factor to stay happy is to cater your worries around, an important relationship in your life and pay special attention sustaining positive relationships. Worries are there to motivate information gathering and problem-solving. Make your mind firm and do come to a positive decision as come what we will not allow the worries to entire our mind and soul. Once a decision is carefully reached we should get busy carrying out our decisions and should not bother about all the anxieties that are about to come. When we, or any of our colleagues or associates, are about to worry about a problem, we must write it out and think positively of the questions: Instead of worrying about what people say of you, why not spend time trying to accomplish something they will admire. What if we just acted like everything was easy? How would your life be different if you stopped worrying about things we can't control and started focusing on the things we can? Let today be the day. You free yourself from fruitless worry, seize the day and take effective action on things you can change. We would change ourselves for the betterment if we start thinking in positive terms. Positive thinking is what is required of us and simply worrying about the future things or as to what will happen in the next moment will certainly deprive us of good and happy living that we are about gather or get in the next hour.

HAPPINESS LIES IN POSITIVE LIVING
BE POSITVE THINK POSITIVE LIVE POSITIVE
CHPTER FORTY

STOP WORRYING?

You may feel largely uncomfortable, when worries attack your thoughts and mind which makes worrying about a situation an easier option to get depressed and diffused. While you are consuming more worries you are far too busy to do anything else to fix the real problem and would rather find it hard to get into a smart solution. Thus resulting in a fact that you spend your evenings worrying only without even bothering to find some time to search a new job. You get nothing out of worrying except only to think and cry. Another cause of getting worried is the attachment with which your inner soul gets attracted to. Attachment brings worry. If you have a problem and you come up with the answer, you stop worrying immediately. Our minds can be dishonest, persuading us that we are worrying about something, when our deepest fear is entirely different. No-one likes to admit that they've chosen to worry. The first step is to write down your worries, which will help you make sense of them, and then decide on one small step you can take towards a solution. But to be very true no man in this world is free of obstacles or difficulties. Don't make worry your habit. Break this habit and stop all the negative and panic thoughts provoking your mind all the time. If you can't change the past, but you must not ruin the present by worrying about the future. Joy is what happens to us when we allow ourselves to recognize how good things really are. When we feel worried and depressed, we need to consciously form a smile on our faces and act upbeat until the

happy feeling becomes genuine reality. Feelings of depression and hopelessness and or anger are even tougher to cope with on a consistent basis. When you are worried, you not only hurt yourself, but the limited support systems that are still holding on your mind but making you to get more and more worried and nothing is achieved in terms of success except the re-carnation of worries and worries your actions breed confidence and courage. If you want to conquer fear, anger and worry do not sit ideal and just think about it. Let our deep worrying become advance thinking and planning.

HAPPINESS LIES IN POSITIVE LIVING
BE POSITVE THINK POSITIVE LIVE POSITIVE
CHAPTER FORTY ONE
FORGET WORRIES

You may feel largely uncomfortable, when worries attack your thoughts and mind which makes worrying about a situation an easier option to get depressed and diffused. While you are consuming more worries you are far too busy to do anything else to fix the real problem and would rather find it hard to get into a smart solution. Thus resulting in a fact that you spend your evenings worrying only without even bothering to find some time to search a new job. You get nothing out of worrying except only to think and cry. Another cause of getting worried is the attachment with which your inner soul gets attracted to. Attachment brings worry. If you have a problem and you come up with the answer, you stop worrying immediately. Our minds can be dishonest, persuading us that we are worrying about something, when our deepest fear is entirely different. No-one likes to admit that they've chosen to worry. The first step is to write down your worries, which will help you make sense of them, and then decide on one small step you can take towards a solution. But to be very true no man in this world is free of obstacles or difficulties. Don't make worry your habit. Break this habit and stop all the negative and panic thoughts provoking your mind all the time. If you can't change the past, but you must not ruin the present by worrying about the future. Joy is what happens to us when we allow ourselves to recognize how good things really are. When we feel worried and depressed, we need to consciously form a smile on our faces and act upbeat until the

happy feeling becomes genuine reality. Feelings of depression and hopelessness and or anger are even tougher to cope with on a consistent basis. When you are worried, you not only hurt yourself, but the limited support systems that are still holding on your mind but making you to get more and more worried and nothing is achieved in terms of success except the re-carnation of worries and worries Your actions breed confidence and courage. If you want to conquer fear, anger and worry do not sit ideal and just think about it. Let our deep worrying become advance thinking and planning. If you look into your own mind and heart, and you find nothing wrong there, what is there to worry about? Practically nothing what is there to fear about and again nothing? So why worry unnecessarily and make your present and future dark. All your thoughts, good and bad, are the creation which tends to lead you to a materialistic life and go in to generate unnecessary worries. That is why you must learn to be more positive. The environment and all the experiences in your life are the results of your habitual and dominant thoughts. Negative thoughts could tell us about something that needs special attention when they lead us to the path of worries. We must discover what needs to be done, and think positively to take care of it. Many of us fail to see a negative occurrence and do not think of a replacement of negative thought with positive one. They even do not look for a bright side in every situation. If we do this for a longer period of time, we become habitual, and it will make a tremendous delay in improving our positive thinking skills. We must remember, everything can be framed positively if we make a restless effort to do so. There are both positive and negative aspects to most situations. We get to choose which ones we will focus on. We can try to catch ourselves when we're being negative and do not try thinking the opposite. There's no sense in worrying about the negatives if these negatives cannot be changed. If we waste energy and happiness on the things we can't change, we'll only make ourselves more frustrated and come to the stage of depression. Negativity is a habit and we often don't realize we're doing ourselves down. Under each negative thought you've written, see if you can spot an alternative way of looking at it, that isn't so negative. There's a world of difference between expecting failure or rejection - so as not to be disappointed when it occurs - and recognizing it as a possibility. It's sensible to look at a situation from all angles and to have a back-up plan to fall back on if need be. People who do this will often see failure as another step on the road to eventual success; but by expecting and envisioning success, there's less likely to be a failure. Let us find some ways of removing negative thoughts and discouraging our worries to be born.

1.   By way of giving a good Smile
The first easiest way is smiling. Many theories have revealed that even a forced smile can lift one's mood. We may also share positivity with others by flashing them with a brilliant smile. Smiling is a reward, not a risk. The only thing we risk when smiling is a giving ourselves a little more happiness.

2.   By way of having the company of good friends.
Keep yourself busy and surround yourself with good friends. Appreciate the people in your life who have stood by you through thick and thin. Count their support which has helped you become more positive, and in the process you will probably help them too. Good friends help each other in the days of crises and through both the good and bad times. Feel positive about them and feel lucky to have them in your company.

3.   Focus your thoughts on positive imagination

Focus your imagination and make efforts on becoming that new positive person. It is much easier to bring about change if you just put your mind to it and change your thoughts into a much more positive direction. We know that it is difficult for us to control things that happen in our lives, but we can, with some effort, control what we think or do in our lives. Positive thinking will make our imagination livelier and we would be able to lead our lives without many worries. Depression, however, has consequences that could ruin your self-esteem, health, and well-being.

HAPPINESS LIES IN POSITIVE LIVING

BE POSITVE THINK POSITIVE LIVE POSITIVE

CHAPTER FORTY TWO

DON'T WORRY -START LIVING

At time we may think that there is no road is left for us from where we can achieve the happiness of our lives. We may also feel that life has become terrible for us to live and we are carrying new hope that someone would come to rescue us. There may be chances that someone who was there with us before might have held on to us when we were on the dark side of the life.

It is important for us to stay open to laughter and humor.

Even when we are facing challenges, it is important for us to stay open to laughter and humor. Sometimes, simply recognizing the potential humor in a situation can lessen our stress and brighten our outlook. Seeking out sources of humor such as watching a funny sitcom or reading jokes online can help us to think more positively. The experience has taught us that we should buy some strength, hope and positive ness from our loved ones to help ourselves in such a situation rather than surrendering as life is a precious gift of God and is equipped with full of joy and happiness if we help ourselves in these critical moments and live with considerable optimism. Happiness in life comes through the doors of positive thoughts; we do not even realize which one is left open.

We have so many reasons to cry and at the same time plenty of reasons to smile as well.

Keeping our dreams and hope alive might be a reason that success and happiness will come our way again. We ought to know that happiness alone does not stand for anything, but it is on our way of thinking that how do we keep ourselves happy in life. Ending up our lives does not lead us to our destination but of course proves we are supposed to be cowards who know not to unfold the doors of belief in God and in ourselves. But if our faith is strong enough we will not be let down, rather we would break the knees of sorrows and force it to die and lead happy lives.

We must find out ways to come out of our worries, anxieties and difficulties.

We should not surrender but must find out ways to come out of our worries, anxieties and difficulties. We ought not to indulge ourselves into the darkness of the room but find out the doors to free ourselves from unnecessary fear and worries. We must belief in ourselves and our hearts, and believe in the ones who love us and not the ones whom we love. We must not fall on the negative side of a thing. It is the real time when we keep on revealing the truth of our lives and relations. We should always try to be happy and should think that whatever is happening, it is the positive side. We should accept the situation and fight it with more determination. We must find out ways to come out of our worries, anxieties and difficulties in order for us to lead a happy sweet and good life.

Negative thoughts are our greatest enemies.

We ought to know that advice from people around us will help us to overcome from the any drastic situation.

Also we have to always minimize the stress as it gives nothing but takes away joy and happiness from our lives. And finally we need to take things casually and fight with it seriously. A clear minded person looks for good qualities in the other person, whereas a negative mind always looks for the fault in the other person, whereas a negative mind always looks for the fault. An optimist goes forward keeping in mind the past, a pessimist thinks of the future and reverts back to the past. In fact negative thoughts are our greatest enemies. Experience the happiness in all circumstances by maintaining better relationships.

We need to analyise the reason for our unhappiness.

Whenever we are unhappy, if we analyze the reason for our unhappiness, it is because life is not matching our desires and expectations. We need to know and realize that nobody is perfect or flawless. If we try to change the way we look, talk and behave just to please others, and show our pride we will gradually become such a person that we ourselves won't recognize each other and would start and create unnecessary worries within us and our surrounding without being positive and will not start to live happily. We ought to stop worrying over unnecessary things be positive and live without fear. Living happily is the master key to all problems and worries. Forgot worries discard all problems take them lightly and behave as nothing serious has happened. This way we are sure to overcome all problems and lead a happy life. We need to understand that what people think of us is their concern, and not ours. If they think about us to be, too reticent or proud, it's really not our business. If every time we happen to meet some new fellows, we may wonder and imagine as what they think of us, and with this feeling in us we will never be able to live a trouble-free and hassle free life. We are bound to fall into the trap of unnecessary worries denying us the startup of new and the happy living life.

Positive attitude is a quality of happy living.

We must think rationally. Is it in our hands or can we control what others think about us? Simply we need to ignore them, if we cannot, and live our lives the way we want to and find the ways to leave worries aside and start living a happy life. Let us make our way to happy living. It is a well-known fact that attitude decides how a natives or persons copes up with the day to day events of life. Attitude is the main influence a person's reaction to a situation in life. It sets the emotional undertone for a person to his likes or dislikes a situation even before he is acquainted with it. Positive attitude is a quality of happy living which is second to none in a human being. We acknowledge our children to say a big thank you from the time to time irrespective they being very little, we teach them to be grateful for everything that they receive. We attach so much importance to this attitude of gratitude that when our children fail to thank someone, we insist that they do it. That is what is needed to be avoided from time to time. We expect this in return from others when we help them or give them a gift. We call a person discourteous and rude when they do not say thank us in return. Though we attach so much importance to this attitude, as we grow into teenage and adult years we find ourselves becoming ungrateful or taking things for granted. We lose touch with the very same qualities that we instill in our children. We take for granted our life, our health, our families, the people in our lives, the things that our loved ones do for us to make our lives easier and things that we possess.

The attitude of positive or happy living speaks a lot about a person.

It denotes about changing negative attitudes and making positive thinking a positive a good habit. Thinking positively and a positive attitude help us to appreciate and value ourselves, our potential and all that we have. It ensures that we do not take our abilities for granted. It makes us look at ourselves as special people with a special set of abilities and potential. It banishes the feelings of inadequacy and insecurity that arises from unfair comparisons with others. It helps us to appreciate people for who they are and not magnify what they are not and their little flaws.

It drives away prejudice and makes us approach life with an open mind. It predisposes us to react to the daily events of life in a positive manner and help us to look at the brighter side of life. Make us optimistic. It gives hope and helps us look forward to life with anticipation making our lives happier and happier day be day. We need to know that positive thinking takes the focus away from what we don't have, to appreciating and making good use of what we have. It is closely connected to our emotional wellbeing and happiness. We feel loved and at peace with ourselves for a major part of our lives when we make this attitude ours. This adds and helps us to get rid of greed, amenity, bitterness, jealousy, and promotes a healthy and nurturing attitude towards others, which in turn gets reciprocated and we feel the sense of healthy living.On the face of it we ought to know that a positive and good living is an attitude that makes you feel good about who you are, what you do, and what your potentials are. This attitude impels you to utilize all that you are endowed with as a person, to achieve the highest possible goals. When we have this attitude, we are able to work without any external pressure to perform but there is sufficient pressure and motivation from within.

Positive thinking and a positive attitude of happy life is a joy for ever

The possessing of happy living is like any other habit, so we need to follow the routine of habit formation here as well. You will win new friends and admirers without having to impress them or conform to the pressure of doing things their way. You will be bubbling with life. You will be rearing to go and accomplish all you can with your new found confidence. The best part of adopting the 'positive thinking and a positive attitude of gratitude is that, you will be able to enjoy the smallest pleasures of nature with a heightened sense of satisfaction and awe. We can see and watch a beautiful flower and carry that joy in our mind for future enjoyment with a clear positive habit. We can go back to work freshen and can use it as an object to meditate on when we feel stressed. When we have this attitude, we are able to work without any external pressure to perform but there is sufficient pressure and motivation from within. The habit of happy living is like any other habit, so we need to follow the routine of habit formation here as well.

Happiness is our own choice and decision. Each of us can be as happy as we make up our minds to be. We can, if we want, fill up our days with positive attitude chatter and laughter. To be happy, we need to concentrate only on happy thoughts. The ghosts of the past have to be exorcised. We may be working in any field, the key to success is our outlook. Sometimes we may think that no road is left for us from where you can achieve the happiness of life. There may be chances that someone who was there with us before might hold on to us when we are on the dark side of the life.

Positive thinking and happy living is state of mind.

Positive thinking and happy living is state of mind and happiness is something we cannot earn or buy. We need to remember that people and things alone, won't make us happy. Our own efforts not to get worried or depressed make us happy. Positive living make us happy. We ought to remember the saying, that "Positive living along can bring happiness as it is a state of mind".

The ultimate goal of life should be to get happiness.

The ultimate goal of life should be to get happiness and not get involved into unnecessary worries falling in the death trap of defeats and failures. The essence of life is not in the great victories and grand failures, but in the simple joys. The purpose of our lives is to be happy. Laugh when we can, apologize when we should, and let go of what we can't change. Let us think positive and just visualize that what is stored in destiny would not be negative. If we want to be happy, practice meditation. If we want, others to be happy practice compassion. Whoever is happy will make others happy, too. Thus we can lead our path to happy sweet and good living.

Our greatest gift to others is to be happy.

Let us be very sure and let us keep in mind that happiness doesn't depend on any superficial conditions, it is governed by our mental attitude only. Our greatest gift to others is to be happy and to radiate our happiness to the entire world. Happiness is a guide to direction, not a place to hide. As a happy person, we radiate happiness to the world. We need to visualize our light radiating throughout the world, passing from person to person until it encircles the globe. Resolve to keep happy, and your joy and you shall form an invincible host against difficulties.

The positive persons often dance to the happy tunes.

The positive persons often dance to the happy tunes of their lives. The path to happiness is forgiveness of everyone and gratitude for everything. Happiness fills your heart each day and your whole life through with clean thoughts. Any day would be a wonderful day if you do not to take life so seriously. Happiness is not about being a winner it is about being gentle with life being gentle within you. Happiness blooms in the presence of self-respect and the absence of ego. Love yourself. Love everyone around you. Love everyone in the whole world.

Happiness is not about being a winner it is about being gentle

When you're feeling depressed or anxious, close your eyes and try to visualize a guided positive imaginary thing. First breathe deeply and relax. How important it is to consistently reach for positive, uplifting, inspirational thoughts. Thought that promote aliveness and abundance. Thoughts that make you feel good. Happiness is not about being a winner it is about being gentle. The only thing between us and our desire, to be happy, is one single fact: we are not happy because we often fall into the death trap of depression and wholly because of our negative thoughts.

Throw away all your negative thoughts.

Throw away all your negative thoughts and worries, concentrate on the goals to be achieved, on the ray of happiness in you and make sure that you are not falling again into the path of negativity. Positive and happy living is not state of mind only it is the discernment of the negatives thoughts .Be a positive thinker and ignore reality in favor of aspirational thoughts. It is more about taking a proactive approach to life. Instead of feeling hopeless or overwhelmed, positive thinking and happy living allows to tackle life's challenges by looking for effective ways to resolve conflict and come up with creative solutions to problems. It might not be easy, but the positive person will surely win and lead a sweet happy and good life.

Happiness in life comes through the doors of positive thoughts;

We do not even realize which one is left open. We have so many reasons to cry and at the same time plenty of reasons to smile as well. Keeping our dreams and hope alive might be a reason that success and happiness will come our way again. We ought to know that happiness alone does not stand for anything, but it is on our way of thinking that how do we keep ourselves happy in life. Ending up our lives does not lead us to our destination but of course proves we are supposed to be cowards who know not to unfold the doors of belief in God and in ourselves.

Failure and disappointment are part of our life.

Failure and disappointment are part of our life. The only thing is that we need to face them boldly and courageously and try our best to solve the problem. We must not forget to believe in God whatever our situation may be we need to make our faith strong enough not be let down, rather we would break the knees of sorrows and force it to die and lead happy lives. We should not surrender but must find out ways to come out of our worries, anxieties and difficulties. We ought not to indulge ourselves into the darkness of the room but find out the doors to free ourselves from unnecessary fear and worries. We must belief in ourselves and our hearts, and believe in the ones who love us and not the ones whom we love. We must not fall on the negative side of a thing.

Happy living is sure to make our life a good and sweet one.

The experience has taught us that we should buy some strength, hope and positive ness from our loved ones to help ourselves in such a situation rather than surrendering our lives to God as it is a precious gift of God which is equipped with full of joy and happiness we need to help ourselves in these critical moments and live with considerable optimism. Happy living is sure to make our life good and sweet. It is the real time when you keep on revealing the truth of our lives and relations, do not fall on the reverse side but think how good it was that because of the hard times of our lives we could well judge about them.

We should always try to be positive and happy

We should always try to be positive and should think that whatever is happening, it is the positive side or consequence of that incident in would be on the positive side of our imagination. With all these thoughts, I would request my readers to implement some good thoughts in their life that would make things easier to be tackled by them. We should accept the situation and fight it with more determination.

In this world nothing is good or bad and only thinking makes it so.

We ought to know that advice from people around us will help us to overcome from the any drastic situation. Also we have to always minimize the stress as it gives nothing but takes away joy and happiness from our lives. And finally we need to take things casually and fight with it seriously. A clear minded person looks for good qualities in the other person, whereas a negative mind always looks for the fault in the other person and also a negative mind always looks for the fault. An optimist goes forward keeping in mind the past, a pessimist thinks of the future and reverts back to the past. In fact negative thoughts are our greatest enemies.

Experience the happiness in all circumstances by maintaining better relationships.

Sadness cannot touch a person with a positive attitude. It increases the decision of making power. Creative way of thoughts appears in the mind. Positive thoughts of happy living teach us the art of finding solutions to any problem. Optimism is something what we do. Anxiety and other negative emotions are known to be detrimental to the body, especially to our immune systems, and having an optimistic nature seems to protect against those effects. People who are supposed to be optimistic, about their future, are sure to lead a sweet good and happy life. Their secret of happiness is that they do exercise, do not indulge in in smoking and often follow a good and better diet. Whenever we are unhappy, if we analyze the reason for our unhappiness, it is because life is not matching our expectations.

HAPPINESS LIES IN POSITIVE LIVING
BE POSITVE THINK POSITIVE LIVE POSITIVE
CHAPTER FORTY THREE

WORRY- LESS AND GET MORE HAPPINESS

If you are interested in getting more success and happiness within you, focus on all the ways as if you have already attained success. You need to focus on the thing and create a happy live within you. If you want love and affection, focus on all the people and the abundance of love that you have to give to them. If we want to have greater health, focus on all the ways that we are healthy, thus creating and delivering a good life within you. You need to admit that there are problems that you cannot change. But you can change the way of your thinking if you identify the main reason of the problem. And if you acknowledge the facts, that you have been negative or inactive in finding a solution to the problem, probably this will make it easier for you to become positive thus creating a new lease of life within you. It will make your life easier to lead a good and sweet life.

You must try to make goals

You must try to make goals. Making goals can give you a more positive outlook on life. People often tend to get bored with life and get the feeling that they are stuck to negative things which the result they often get the feeling of being depressed. Setting a direction for yourself and a goal would surely help you to move forward.

Mental attitude that can bring you peace and happiness

If you expecting to succeed, and are not afraid of failure, you have the best chance of staying positive and can create a very positive life within you. When you, or any of your associates, are tempted to worry about a problem, write out the solution and a definite answer to it. This helps a positive feeling to generate within you making you very positive to have a good living. Another thing you need to understand is that there are several ways to cultivate a mental attitude that can bring you peace and happiness and can carnage a good life within you. More of it if you fill your mind with thoughts of peace, courage, health, and hope, your life will be easy to live. You would get a happy feeling of life and mind if you let yourself to forget your own unhappiness, by trying to create a little happiness for others. You are best to yourself and to others.

The first step is to write down your worries

The first step is to write down your worries, which will help you make sense of them, and then decide on one small step you can take towards a solution. But to be very true no man in this world is free of obstacles or difficulties. Don't make worry your habit. Break this habit and stop all the negative and panic thoughts provoking your mind all the time. If you can't change the past, but you must not ruin the present by worrying about the future. Joy is what happens to us when we allow ourselves to recognize how good things really are. When we feel worried and depressed, we need to consciously form a smile on our faces and act upbeat until the happy feeling becomes genuine reality.

Happiness is what is needed most.

What makes to lead a happy life is not to get trapped into unnecessary unwanted worries and negative thoughts. Don't create the feeling of depression and anger. Feelings of depression and hopelessness and or anger are even tougher to cope with on a consistent basis. When you are worried, you not only hurt yourself, but the limited support systems that are still holding on your mind but making you to get more and more worried and nothing is achieved in terms of success except the re-carnation of worries and worries thus leading you to be unhappy and worried all the time. Your actions breed confidence and courage. If you want to conquer fear, anger and worry do not sit ideal and just think about it. Let our deep worrying become advance thinking and planning. If you look into your own mind and heart, and you find nothing wrong there, what is there to worry about? Practically nothing what is there to fear about and again nothing? So why worry unnecessarily and make your present and future dark. Neglect all those which make your life unhappy.

Why being a negative person?

Why being a negative person and what do you get out of it being a depression dejected and sad man.? Why not turn your thoughts to be a positive person simply it is a question of tilting your mind towards a positive side of thing. See both the aspects of a situation and ways the pros and cons of both the sides and try to abolish the negativity in you. Be positive strong and you will remain happy for ever. We all have different roles that we play in the lives of people we love and care about. Our actions and how well we play our part has a direct influence on their life, so we better get in there and give our best performance. Tell them with how much you care in the capacity that you're in. At the end of the day, money is just a means to an end. Nothing more. If you're grinding and struggling to make ends meet and buried under piles of debt, that's pretty stressful. Once you have your basic needs met though, more money only makes you happier up to a certain point. Money cannot buy you happiness. You need to generate it yourself. Someone will always be better than you at something, but it does not matter. Be inspired by them, using it to push yourself further, and nothing more. If they can do it, why cannot you? If you are interested in getting more happiness focus on all the ways as if you have already attained success. You need to focus on the thing and create a live within you. If you want love and affection, focus on all the people and the abundance of love that you have to give to them.

Worrisome thoughts reproduce faster.

Worrisome thoughts reproduce faster so one of the most powerful ways to stop the spiral of worry is simply to disclose the worry to a friend. Practice happy gratitude daily. Take three minutes at the end of your day to chill and write down a small list of the things that can make you smile, laugh, or that you're glad are a part of your life. There's something to be grateful about, especially when you look down at that list and realize that a lot of people have it worse off than you do and could use a few of those things. Simply being an optimist will not solve all your problems, but what's the alternative is to keep your mind and heart cool and always have happy and positive feeling and think that life is to live happily. There isn't much sense in being anything else. If you're constantly filling your head with negative thoughts, odds are they'll lead you straight towards negative actions, self-doubt and increase the general happiness of life isn't a cool place to live at all.

What do we get out of unhappiness?

We may feel largely uncomfortable, when worries attack our thoughts and mind. While we are consuming more worries we are far too busy to do anything else to fix the real problem and would rather find it hard to get into a smart solution. Thus resulting in a fact that you spend your evenings worrying only without even bothering to find some time to know its cause We get nothing out of worrying except only to think and cry and become unhappy. We do not get anything out of unhappiness. Another thing is that we may feel largely uncomfortable, when worries attack our thoughts and mind which makes worrying about a situation an easier option to get depressed and diffused. While we are consuming more worries we are far too busy to do anything else to fix the real problem and would rather find it hard to get into a smart solution. Thus resulting in a fact that we spend our evenings worrying only without even bothering to find some time to search a sweet happiness within us.

Negative thoughts create unnecessary worries

Negative thought which are provoking our mind, about the uncertainties and the negativities, as to what will happen tomorrow creates unnecessary worries and worries are repetitive thoughts associated with feelings of anxiety in anticipation of some negative future event which may end in a failure. Whether the worries are about financial crisis, family problems, work, health or any topic of concern, the anxious feelings and negative thoughts produced are always distinctly unpleasant thus making us unhappy all the time. We get nothing being a negative and unhappy man. We must not forget that if we tend to worry they will never rob tomorrow of its sorrows, but will only deny today of its meaning happiness and joys. Negative thoughts only produce worries and worrying is actually a form of superstition and creates false images in our mind and that is the main reason and cause which makes and leads us to this point of imagination. A human being can survive almost anything, as long as he or she sees the end in sight, starts analyzing his positive thoughts and starts analyzing his unhappiness.

We need to fore see the coming trouble first.

We must not forgot that if something bad or good is to happen it is sure to happen, whether we worry or not. Let us put our energy into today and stop worrying about the future and past. We should not foresee trouble, or worry about what may never happen as past is dead and gone forever and future is uncertain and yet to come. Positive thinking our brave attitude and our courage will ward off everything and bring happiness in our lives. The basic facts we should know about worry. The basic techniques to analyze worry and how to break the worry habit before it breaks us. These are the simple ways where we can concentrate and get rid of worries prevailing in our thoughts, remove all the negativity in our live and start living a positive good and happy life.

Think of good and positive ways of Happy Living.

Annalise positive ways of happy living and get to see the reasons and facts of worry. To avoid reoccurrence of worries, concentrate on prayers as prayers are the best source of remedies of the prevailing worries. Think good ways of living and starting praying. The more you pray, the less you'll panic. The more you worship, the less you worry. There is nothing that wastes the body like worry, and anyone who has any faith in God should need not to worry about anything whatsoever is to happen in future. Positive thinking is the creation of good imagination and good imagination is the creation of sweet and happy living.

Happiness comes with Positive living and sweet thoughts

If you know that the circumstance is beyond your control or power change than revise it to your liking. Just try to put a stop-less order on your worries. Don't permit little things which become insects of life to ruin your happiness. Co-operate with the inevitable. Decide just how much anxiety a thing may be worth and refuse to give in anymore.

All the happiness is not given in one go it comes slowly and slowly with positive thinking.

Have worry under your control. If your worries center around, pay special attention to remain positive and be happy. Keep yourself happy, treat your worried thoughts as valuable signals. How to keep from worrying about criticism? Simply unjust criticism and think positively and do often discard a bad compliment. It often means that you have aroused jealousy and envy. Let's keep a record of the fool things we have done and stop criticizing ourselves.

Cause of unhappiness is Negative way of living life

The utmost cause of worry is our negative thinking as it leads us to the state of depression. Living will change for the better-If You Think Positive. Our negative thinking and attitude towards suffering and depression becomes very important because it can affect how we cope with suffering when it arises. Depression is nourished by a lifetime of un-grieved and unforgiven causes. Times will change for the better when you change. Worry is a misuse of the imagination. Worry is most often a prideful way of thinking that you have more control over life and its circumstances than you actually do. Positive Thinking leads your way to good and happiness. An art of Good and Happy Living.

Neglect worries keep yourself happy.

Neglect worries keep yourself happy, treat your worried thoughts as valuable signals. These are the fundamental facts you should be familiar about worries. A huge factor to stay happy is to cater your worries around, an important relationship in your life and pay special attention sustaining positive relationships. Worries are there to motivate information gathering and problem-solving. Make your mind firm and do come to a positive decision as come what we will not allow the worries to entire our mind and soul.

What if we just acted like everything was easy?

Once a decision is carefully reached we should get busy carrying out our decisions and should not bother about all the anxieties that are about to come. When we, or any of our colleagues or associates, are about to worry about a problem, we must write it out and think positively of the questions. Instead of worrying about what people say of you, why not spend time trying to accomplish something they will admire. What if we just acted like everything was easy? How would your life be different if you stopped worrying about things we can't control and started focusing on the things we can? Let today be the day.

Free yourself from fruitless worry, seize the day and take effective action on things you can change. We would change ourselves for the betterment if we start thinking in positive terms. Positive thinking is what is required of us and simply worrying about the future things or as to what will happen in the next moment will certainly deprive us of good and happy living that we are about gather or get in the next hour.

Another cause of getting worried or unhappy is the attachment

Attachment brings worry. If you have a problem and you come up with the answer, you stop worrying immediately. Our minds can be dishonest, persuading us that we are worrying about something, when our deepest fear is entirely different. No-one likes to admit that they've chosen to worry. The first step is to write down your worries, which will help you make sense of them, and then decide on one small step you can take towards a solution. But to be very true no man in this world is free of obstacles or difficulties. Don't make worry your habit. Break this habit and stop all the negative and panic thoughts provoking your mind all the time if you want to remain a happy person and lead a happy good and sweet life. Feelings of depression and angry are even tougher to cope with on a consistent basis. When you are worried, you not only hurt yourself, but the limited support systems that are still holding on your mind making you to get more and more worried and nothing is achieved in terms of success except the re-carnation of worries and worries Joy is what happens to us when we allow ourselves to recognize how good things really are.

Practically nothing what is there to fear about?

So why worry unnecessarily and make your present and future dark. Why being a negative person and what do you get out of it being a depression dejected and sad man.? Why not turn your thoughts to be a positive person simply it is a question of tilting your mind towards a positive side of thing. See both the aspects of a situation and ways the pros and cons of both the sides and try to abolish the negativity in you. You will surely be a happy man.

Think of the best the best is sure to happen

Think of the best the best is sure to happen and if you think of the worst the worst will come. Better come forward wake up and think positive first. Positive persons always succeed in life whatever be the circumstances and the negative often dig a death trap for themselves. So why be a negative person why you have all the qualities of being a positive man. Surround yourself with friends and people that are better than you in areas that you want to improve in. Even when you are facing challenges, it is important to stay open to laughter and humor. Sometimes, simply recognizing the potential humor in a situation can lessen your stress and brighten your outlook. Seeking out sources of humor such as watching a funny sitcom or reading jokes online can help you think more positive thoughts. We need to know and realize that nobody is perfect or flawless. If we try to change the way we look, talk and behave just to please others, and show our pride we will gradually become such a person that we ourselves won't recognize each other and would start and create unnecessary worries within us and our surrounding without being positive and will not start to live happily. We ought to stop worrying over unnecessary things be positive and live without fear happily. As a result, negative thoughts can creep into your mind. While you know that thinking positively is better for your state of mind, you might be surprised to learn that it can also be good for your health. We need to understand that what people think of us is their concern, and not ours. If they think about us to be, too reticent or proud, it's really not our business. If every time we happen to meet some new fellows, we may wonder and imagine as what they think of us, and with this feeling in us we will never be able to live a trouble-free and hassle free life. We are bound to fall into the trap of unnecessary worries denying us the startup of new and the happy living life. We must think rationally. Is it in our hands or can we control what others think about us? Simply we need to ignore them If we cannot, and live our lives the way we want to and find the ways to leave worries aside and start living a happy life. Let us make our way to happy living.

Positive Thinking with Positive Attitudes.

Positive thinking is not about putting on a pair of rose-colored glasses and ignoring all the negative things you will encounter in life. That approach can be just as devastating as ignoring the positive and only focusing on the negative. Balance, with a healthy dose of realism, is the key. It is a well-known fact that attitude decides how a natives or persons copes up with the day to day events of life. Attitude is what a influence a person's reaction to a situation in life is. It sets the emotional undertone for a person to his likes or dislikes a situation even before he is acquainted with it. Positive attitude is a quality that is second to none in a human being. Though we attach so much importance to this attitude, as we grow into teenage and adult years we find ourselves becoming ungrateful or taking things for granted. We lose touch with the very same qualities that we instill in our children. We take for granted our life, our health, our families, the people in our lives, the things that our loved ones do for us to make our lives easier and things that we possess. The attitude of positive speaks a lot about a person. It denotes about changing negative attitudes and making positive thinking a positive attitude a good habit. Thinking positively and a positive attitude help us to appreciate and value ourselves, our potential and all that we have. It ensures that we do not take our abilities for granted. It makes us look at ourselves as special people with a special set of abilities and potential. It banishes the feelings of inadequacy and insecurity that arises from unfair comparisons with others. It helps us to appreciate people for who they are and not magnify what they are not and their little flaws. It drives away prejudice and makes us approach life with an open mind. It predisposes us to react to the daily events of life in a positive manner and help us to look at the brighter side of life. Make us optimistic. It gives hope and helps us look forward to life with anticipation. We need to know that positive thinking takes the focus away from what we don't have, to appreciating and making good use of what we have. It is closely connected to our emotional wellbeing and happiness. We feel loved and at peace with ourselves for a major part of our lives when we make this attitude ours. This adds and helps us to get rid of greed, amenity, bitterness, jealousy, and promotes a healthy and nurturing attitude towards others, which in turn gets reciprocated and we feel the sense of healthy living. We attach so much importance to this attitude of gratitude that when our children fail to thank someone, we insist that they do it. That is what is needed to be avoided from time to time. We expect this in return from others when we help them or give them a gift. We call a person discourteous and rude when they do not say thank us in return. On the face of it we ought to know that a positive is not an attitude of being satisfied and content, that you never want to do anything, anymore.

This is an attitude that makes you feel good about who you are, what you do, and what your potentials are. This attitude impels you to utilize all that you are endowed with as a person, to achieve the highest possible goals. When we have this attitude, we are able to work without any external pressure to perform but there is sufficient pressure and motivation from within. The possessing of positive thinking is like any other habit, so we need to follow the routine of habit formation here as well. You will win new friends and admirers without having to impress them or conform to the pressure of doing things their way. You will be bubbling with life and the joie de vivre. You will be rearing to go and accomplish all you can with your new found confidence. The best part of adopting the 'positive thinking and a positive attitude of gratitude is that, you will be able to enjoy the smallest pleasures of nature with a heightened sense of satisfaction and awe. I can see and watch a beautiful flower and carry that joy in my mind for future enjoyment with a clear positive habit. I can go back to work freshen and can use it as an object to meditate on when I feel stressed. Let us be clear that a positive is not an attitude of being satisfied and content, that you never want to do anything, anymore. This is an attitude that makes you feel good about who you are, what you do, and what your potentials are. This attitude impels you to utilize all that you are endowed with as a person, to achieve the highest possible goals. When we have this attitude, we are able to work without any external pressure to perform but there is sufficient pressure and motivation from within. The habit of positive thinking is like any other habit, so we need to follow the routine of habit formation here as well. We should always remember that, "Life is there, where there is hope". That single thing that remains in our hands is to find out ways to know how to overcome these worries of our life at that very moment when all doors are closed for us which means that whatever situation is there, we must not give up hope. We must fight because there have been always a chance that with good faith and hard work we can turn the odds in our favor. is often said that it is very easy to advice but when it comes to us, things go out of our control and we fail to suggest a way out for ourselves. We fall into the trap of unnecessary worries and elope ourselves negative thoughts. We feel better when somebody else is facing some difficulty but when it comes to us we fail to gather that faith, will power and the words of strength. Being a positive thinker is not about ignoring reality in favor of aspirational thoughts. It is more about taking a proactive approach to your life. Instead of feeling hopeless or overwhelmed, positive thinking allows you to tackle life's challenges by looking for effective ways to resolve conflict and come up with creative solutions to problems. It might not be easy, but the positive impact it will have on your mental, emotional, and physical health will be well-worth it. It takes practice; lots of practice.

This is not a step-by-step process that you can complete and be done with. Instead, it involves a lifelong commitment to looking inside yourself and being willing to challenge negative thoughts and make positive changes. It is a common fact that no one in this world is free of obstacles or difficulties. If all the openings of happiness are shut for us and we have to overcome that and have no way to come out, but to survive lest we must have to learn to swim out of the sorrows because this is what is called life and sorrow free living. There are lot more examples and in many other situations, where we will find that how we could have faced and fought with our sorrows and difficulties of life when there was no hope left in our lives. When the power of will is at the worst and each one of us knows that the one who is gone never comes back. Neither a thousands of words would not be enough to bring him back nor a million tears, because each and every moment, eyes would only shed tears , mind would remain tensed and we would be simply surrounded by worries and the life seems to have been vanished. Life is ever expanding, contraction is death. As commonly said by big saints that the self- seeking man who is looking after his personal comforts and leading a lazy life for himself there would be no room for him even in the hell and he simply have lost the power of his will. One cannot do anything without it. We fail only when we do not try very hard to achieve the power and faith within us. As soon as we lose faith, death comes in our way and we are surrounds by all the evils and stupid worries of the world. The secret and history of every successful man is to have, good confidence, faith and strength behind him and that remain the right cause of his single success in life. Unselfishness plays a very vital role in his life. He may not have been perfectly unselfish, yet he was tending towards it. If he had been perfectly unselfish, he would have been as great a success. The degree of unselfishness marks the degree of success everywhere and he leads to be successful man without fear worries and selfishness. Therefore creation of positivity in life is utmost necessary to enjoy the special gift of God to us. The love for God and worshipping God adds to one common thing the immense faith in Him. There may be different beliefs and ways to worship God in different communities, places and religions, but one thing remains the same and that is the Love of God for all of us. Our world is full of odds and evens, happiness and sorrows, fulfilment and emptiness. And these are all created by the Almighty. However, the most beautiful Gift of God, is Human, which is such a mystery driven by Him which could hardly be defined or explained in depth. We know that life cannot be foreseen. Life is not a bed of roses. Life is a battle field and not a bed of roses as every man on earth has to struggle very hard in making his life happy. If aim of our life is to stay happy and let others to be happy, we will be happy and remembered by all. But no one will actually remember us for the wealth we have gained, or success we have achieved. I have no aim in life. Summary living with no purpose in life is just like a feather moving towards the wind. Life is such a special gift of Almighty and it is not gifted by Him to use it the way we like or love to. The actual path shown by Him needs to be followed by us for us to reach the peak of betterment every moment. We need to have some positive attitude to look at it comfortably but at the same time having a positive mental attitude does not mean banishing all negative thoughts and people from your life. One and another one arises.

Negative thoughts create unnecessary worries

Whether the worries are about financial crisis, family problems, work, health or any topic of concern, the anxious feelings and negative thoughts produced are always distinctly unpleasant thus making us unhappy all the time. We get nothing being a negative and unhappy man. We must not forget that if we tend to worry they will never rob tomorrow of its sorrows, but will only deny today of its meaning happiness and joys. Negative thoughts only produce worries and worrying is actually a form of superstition and creates false images in our mind and that is the main reason and cause which makes and leads us to this point of imagination. A human being can survive almost anything, as long as he or she sees the end in sight, starts analyzing his positive thoughts and starts analyzing his unhappiness.

HAPPINESS LIES IN POSITIVE LIVING

BE POSITVE THINK POSITIVE LIVE POSITIVE

CHAPTER FORTY FOUR

STOP WORRYING AND START LIVING

At time we may think that there is no road is left for us from where we can achieve the happiness of our lives. We may also feel that life has become terrible for us to live and we are carrying new hope that someone would come to rescue us. There may be chances that someone who was there with us before might have held on to us when we were on the dark side of the life.

It is important for us to stay open to laughter and humor.

Even when we are facing challenges, it is important for us to stay open to laughter and humor. Sometimes, simply recognizing the potential humor in a situation can lessen our stress and brighten our outlook. Seeking out sources of humor such as watching a funny sitcom or reading jokes online can help us to think more positively. The experience has taught us that we should buy some strength, hope and positive ness from our loved ones to help ourselves in such a situation rather than surrendering as life is a precious gift of God and is equipped with full of joy and happiness if we help ourselves in these critical moments and live with considerable optimism. Happiness in life comes through the doors of positive thoughts; we do not even realize which one is left open.

We have so many reasons to cry and at the same time plenty of reasons to smile as well.

Keeping our dreams and hope alive might be a reason that success and happiness will come our way again. We ought to know that happiness alone does not stand for anything, but it is on our way of thinking that how do we keep ourselves happy in life. Ending up our lives does not lead us to our destination but of course proves we are supposed to be cowards who know not to unfold the doors of belief in God and in ourselves. But if our faith is strong enough we will not be let down, rather we would break the knees of sorrows and force it to die and lead happy lives.

We must find out ways to come out of our worries, anxieties and difficulties.

We should not surrender but must find out ways to come out of our worries, anxieties and difficulties. We ought not to indulge ourselves into the darkness of the room but find out the doors to free ourselves from unnecessary fear and worries. We must belief in ourselves and our hearts, and believe in the ones who love us and not the ones whom we love. We must not fall on the negative side of a thing. It is the real time when we keep on revealing the truth of our lives and relations. We should always try to be happy and should think that whatever is happening, it is the positive side. We should accept the situation and fight it with more determination. We must find out ways to come out of our worries, anxieties and difficulties in order for us to lead a happy sweet and good life.

Negative thoughts are our greatest enemies.

We ought to know that advice from people around us will help us to overcome from the any drastic situation. Also we have to always minimize the stress as it gives nothing but takes away joy and happiness from our lives. And finally we need to take things casually and fight with it seriously. A clear minded person looks for good qualities in the other person, whereas a negative mind always looks for the fault in the other person, whereas a negative mind always looks for the fault. An optimist goes forward keeping in mind the past, a pessimist thinks of the future and reverts back to the past. In fact negative thoughts are our greatest enemies. Experience the happiness in all circumstances by maintaining better relationships.

We need to analyise the reason for our unhappiness.

Whenever we are unhappy, if we analyze the reason for our unhappiness, it is because life is not matching our desires and expectations. We need to know and realize that nobody is perfect or flawless. If we try to change the way we look, talk and behave just to please others, and show our pride we will gradually become such a person that we ourselves won't recognize each other and would start and create unnecessary worries within us and our surrounding without being positive and will not start to live happily. We ought to stop worrying over unnecessary things be positive and live without fear. Living happily is the master key to all problems and worries. Forgot worries discard all problems take them lightly and behave as nothing serious has happened. This way we are sure to overcome all problems and lead a happy life. We need to understand that what people think of us is their concern, and not ours. If they think about us to be, too reticent or proud, it's really not our business. If every time we happen to meet some new fellows, we may wonder and imagine as what they think of us, and with this feeling in us we will never be able to live a trouble-free and hassle free life. We are bound to fall into the trap of unnecessary worries denying us the startup of new and the happy living life.

Positive attitude is a quality of happy living.

We must think rationally. Is it in our hands or can we control what others think about us? Simply we need to ignore them, if we cannot, and live our lives the way we want to and find the ways to leave worries aside and start living a happy life. Let us make our way to happy living. It is a well-known fact that attitude decides how a natives or persons copes up with the day to day events of life. Attitude is the main influence a person's reaction to a situation in life. It sets the emotional undertone for a person to his likes or dislikes a situation even before he is acquainted with it. Positive attitude is a quality of happy living which is second to none in a human being. We acknowledge our children to say a big thank you from the time to time irrespective they being very little, we teach them to be grateful for everything that they receive. We attach so much importance to this attitude of gratitude that when our children fail to thank someone, we insist that they do it. That is what is needed to be avoided from time to time. We expect this in return from others when we help them or give them a gift. We call a person discourteous and rude when they do not say thank us in return. Though we attach so much importance to this attitude, as we grow into teenage and adult years we find ourselves becoming ungrateful or taking things for granted. We lose touch with the very same qualities that we instill in our children. We take for granted our life, our health, our families, the people in our lives, the things that our loved ones do for us to make our lives easier and things that we possess.

The attitude of positive or happy living speaks a lot about a person.

It denotes about changing negative attitudes and making positive thinking a positive a good habit. Thinking positively and a positive attitude help us to appreciate and value ourselves, our potential and all that we have. It ensures that we do not take our abilities for granted. It makes us look at ourselves as special people with a special set of abilities and potential. It banishes the feelings of inadequacy and insecurity that arises from unfair comparisons with others. It helps us to appreciate people for who they are and not magnify what they are not and their little flaws. It drives away prejudice and makes us approach life with an open mind. It predisposes us to react to the daily events of life in a positive manner and help us to look at the brighter side of life. Make us optimistic. It gives hope and helps us look forward to life with anticipation making our lives happier and happier day by day. We need to know that positive thinking takes the focus away from what we don't have, to appreciating and making good use of what we have. It is closely connected to our emotional wellbeing and happiness. We feel loved and at peace with ourselves for a major part of our lives when we make this attitude ours. This adds and helps us to get rid of greed, amenity, bitterness, jealousy, and promotes a healthy and nurturing attitude towards others, which in turn gets reciprocated and we feel the sense of healthy living. On the face of it we ought to know that a positive and good living is an attitude that makes you feel good about who you are, what you do, and what your potentials are. This attitude impels you to utilize all that you are endowed with as a person, to achieve the highest possible goals. When we have this attitude, we are able to work without any external pressure to perform but there is sufficient pressure and motivation from within.

Positive thinking and a positive attitude of happy life is a joy for ever

The possessing of happy living is like any other habit, so we need to follow the routine of habit formation here as well. You will win new friends and admirers without having to impress them or conform to the pressure of doing things their way. You will be bubbling with life. You will be rearing to go and accomplish all you can with your new found confidence. The best part of adopting the 'positive thinking and a positive attitude of gratitude is that, you will be able to enjoy the smallest pleasures of nature with a heightened sense of satisfaction and awe. We can see and watch a beautiful flower and carry that joy in our mind for future enjoyment with a clear positive habit. We can go back to work freshen and can use it as an object to meditate on when we feel stressed.

HAPPINESS LIES IN POSITIVE LIVING

BE POSITVE THINK POSITIVE LIVE POSITIVE

CHAPTER FORTY FIVE

WHY NOT LIVE HAPPILY AND SWEETLY

Thought which are provoking our mind, about the uncertainties and the negativities, as to what will happen tomorrow. Worries that are prevailing in our minds are repetitive thoughts associated with feelings of anxiety in anticipation of some negative future event. Whether the worries are about financial crisis, family problems, work, health or any topic of concern, the anxious feelings produced and sustained by the imaginary thoughts which always distinctly appear to be unpleasant. Positive Thinking leads us to a happy life one must not forgot the life is what we make it, so let us make it a happy one! Don't worry on things that may not happen, life is too short to worry too much. Smile and be happy. Make yourself to be positive person.Keep smiling in the sunlight. Imagine every day to be a positive day and the last of a life surrounded with hopes, the hours that come unexpectedly will be much the more grateful. The mind that is anxious about future events is miserable. Present fears are less than horrible imaginings. Positive thinking is sure to ward of every odd imagination and sure to make you a happy person. Happy living actually means approaching life's challenges with a positive outlook. It does not necessarily mean avoiding or ignoring the bad things; instead, it involves making the most of potentially bad situations, trying to see the best in other people, and viewing yourself and your abilities in a positive light. Happy living centers on such things as a belief in abilities, a positive approach to challenges, and trying to make the most of bad situations. Bad things will happen. Sometimes you will be disappointed or hurt by the actions of others. This does not mean that the world is out to get you or that all people will let you down. Instead, happy living will look at the situation realistically, search for ways that they can improve the situation, and try to learn from their experiences. Happy living brings good cheer, remembering that the misfortunes hardest to bear are those that never happen, focus on the positive aspects of lives, rather than on the negative setbacks. Let us not waste our lives in doubts and fears. It is not work that kills us, it is worry and the negative thinking. Work is healthy; but worry is rust upon the blade. It is not movement that destroys the machinery, but friction. We need to forget the most disturbing negative thinking in our lives and opt for the positive attitude by following the principles of happy living. Not only can happy living impact our ability to cope with stress and our immunity, it also has an impact on our overall well-being. Our success lies only in our happy living. Look to be happy think in positive terms and think as if the unhappiness is not there at lot and God has given us this precious life to enjoy to our fullest all the fruits of happiness of our lives. Happy living and good living is definitely an "Art of Sweet Living".

CREATE HAPPINESS WITHIN YOU

If you are interested in getting more happiness, to get it through positive thinking. all you need to do is to focus on all the directions on positive thinking as if you have already attained success. You need to focus on the thing and create a life within you. If you want love and affection, entertain people and give them the abundance of love. If you want to have greater health, pay attention on all the ways that make us healthy, thus creating and delivering a good life within you by thinking in positive ways. You need to understand and admit that there are problems that you cannot change. But you can change the ways of your thinking if you identify the main reason of the problem. And if you acknowledge the facts, that you have been negative or inactive in finding a solution to the problem, probably this will make it easier for you to become positive thus creating a new lease of life within you. Positive thinking will surely make you happy. Another thing to understand is that you must try to make goals. Making goals can give you a more positive outlook on life. People often tend to get bored with life and get the feeling that they are stuck to negative things with the result they often get the feeling of being depressed dejected and monotonous. Setting a direction and a goal for yourself, would surely help you to move forward. If you are expecting to succeed, and are not afraid of failure, you have the best chance of staying positive and can create a very positive life within you. When you, or any of your associates, are tempted to worry about a problem, write out the solution and a definite answer to it. This helps a positive feeling to generate within you.

The perfect way to conquer worry is the Prayer of God

Another thing you need to understand is that there are several ways to cultivate a mental attitude that can bring you peace and happiness and can carnage a good life within you. More of it if you fill your mind with thoughts of peace, courage, health, and hope, your life will be easy to live. If you think in positive terms you would get a happy feeling of life and mind you if you let yourself to forget your own unhappiness, by trying to create a little happiness for others you are sure to get happiness in your live. You are best to yourself. The perfect way to conquer worry is the Prayer of God. To keep yourself from worrying about criticism, do not even try to get mixed with your enemies, because if you do you will hurt yourself far more than we hurting them. You will fall prey to negative thinking and this in turn will lead you unhappiness in life. Instead of worrying about ingratitude, let's expect it. Let's remember that the only way to find happiness is not to expect gratitude, but to give for the joy of giving. Let us build a happy life within us generate peace and a healthy atmosphere around us. This will help us to lead a peaceful happy and prosperous life and we would find ourselves to be happier than before. You should do things in the order of their importance. If you have or face problems in hand you need to clear your desk of all papers except those relating to the immediate problem at hand. When you face a problem, solve it then and there, by thinking positively and if you have the facts to make a decision, make a decision fast and do not linger on. Learn to think in positive terms organize the things, deputize, and supervise straight away by coming to decision. Simply postponing it would spoil your good thoughts and there is every likelihood your mind may get into negative activities and start thinking in negative manner. Therefore think positive, write down a list of things that make you positive, however big, small, likely or unlikely. Then work to make them occur more often. Look for moments of joy and savor them. Recognize your good happening every day. Be positive think positive and be happy.

Take care of your health- Eat Well

One need not to forgot that we need to eat well do plenty of exercise and do not skip meals It is a known fact that physical exercise is known to stimulate our veins and get to strengthen our minds that lift depression and anxiety, so we need to walk, swim, run or whatever we like doing best above all we must move ahead in direction where our mind can generate electricity to think in positive direct. So take care of your health and eat well. Those who create negativity or those who not well tend to give themselves worry and stress and in the end tend to be devastated. If we cannot get some good sunshine, we can always lighten up our thoughts with brighter lights of positive thinking. We can have ample of lunch of positive thinking. To avoid negative thoughts we need to take frequent walks No man is indispensable and no man is not capable of positive thinking. Our friends are always there to give us some moral support. Spending time and engaging ourselves in worthwhile positive activities could give us a very enjoyable and satisfying feeling. Nothing feels better than having group support and talking in terms of positive thinking. Good friends are quite important and their company generally lightened up our spirits. This makes us to think in positive manner and to get to know such friends we simply have to be friendly with ourselves, and then the friendships will naturally follow us and make our lives happy. We need to understand the power of positive thinking and its support and we have not to underestimate it strength and support. Don't we feel so good when someone pats us on our back and gives us some words of encouragement during your most challenging times and difficult times and advises us to remain positive and think positive just hug or embrace someone with positive attitude someday you will see that you have almost changed his life. Get intimate with him and try to establish close ties with his family and friends. The love and care expressed by you will tremendously boost him in positive manner and well as your immune system and fury of worry will be diminished for all if you advise them to think in positive terms. In our lives difficulties and storms may come and go in the form of reversals, but if we have the power of positive thinking and foundation of inner fulfillment we would be able to deal with it with a very clear practical mind and with this positive thinking these storms will not kill us nor will disrupt us. There could be numberless reasons for which we keep on worrying. We may be worried about our health, wealth, loved ones, friends, the happening of yesterday and the follow happenings of tomorrow, the environment or the world politics, but these can be dealt with firm mind and fearless worry if we generate within ourselves the power of positive thinking within ourselves.

HAPPINESS LIES IN POSITIVE LIVING

BE POSITVE THINK POSITIVE LIVE POSITIVE

CHAPTER FORTY SIX

START HAPPY LIVING

Even when you are facing challenges, it is important to stay open to laughter and humor. Sometimes, simply recognizing the potential humor in a situation can lessen your stress and brighten your outlook. Seeking out sources of humor such as watching a funny sitcom or reading jokes online can help you think more positive thoughts. We need to know and realize that nobody is perfect or flawless. If we try to change the way we look, talk and behave just to please others, and show our pride we will gradually become such a person that we ourselves won't recognize each other and would start and create unnecessary worries within us and our surrounding without being positive and will not start to live happily. We ought to stop worrying over unnecessary things be positive and live without fear happily. As a result, negative thoughts can creep into your mind. While you know that thinking positively is better for your state of mind, you might be surprised to learn that it can also be good for your health. We need to understand that what people think of us is their concern, and not ours. If they think about us to be, too reticent or proud, it's really not our business. If every time we happen to meet some new fellows, we may wonder and imagine as what they think of us, and with this feeling in us we will never be able to live a trouble-free and hassle free life. We are bound to fall into the trap of unnecessary worries denying us the startup of new and the happy living life. We must think rationally. Is it in our hands or can we control what others think about us?. Simply we need to ignore them If we cannot, and live our lives the way we want to and find the ways to leave worries aside and start living a happy life. Let us make our way to happy living.

Positive Thinking with Positive Attitudes.

Positive thinking is not about putting on a pair of rose-colored glasses and ignoring all the negative things you will encounter in life. That approach can be just as devastating as ignoring the positive and only focusing on the negative. Balance, with a healthy dose of realism, is the key. It is a well-known fact that attitude decides how a natives or persons copes up with the day to day events of life. Attitude is what a influence a person's reaction to a situation in life is. It sets the emotional undertone for a person to his likes or dislikes a situation even before he is acquainted with it. Positive attitude is a quality that is second to none in a human being. Though we attach so much importance to this attitude, as we grow into teenage and adult years we find ourselves becoming ungrateful or taking things for granted. We lose touch with the very same qualities that we instill in our children. We take for granted our life, our health, our families, the people in our lives, the things that our loved ones do for us to make our lives easier and things that we possess. The attitude of positive speaks a lot about a person. It denotes about changing negative attitudes and making positive thinking a positive attitude a good habit. Thinking positively and a positive attitude help us to appreciate and value ourselves, our potential and all that we have. It ensures that we do not take our abilities for granted. It makes us look at ourselves as special people with a special set of abilities and potential. It banishes the feelings of inadequacy and insecurity that arises from unfair comparisons with others. It helps us to appreciate people for who they are and not magnify what they are not and their little flaws. It drives away prejudice and makes us approach life with an open mind. It predisposes us to react to the daily events of life in a positive manner and help us to look at the brighter side of life. Make us optimistic. It gives hope and helps us look forward to life with anticipation. We need to know that positive thinking takes the focus away from what we don't have, to appreciating and making good use of what we have. It is closely connected to our emotional wellbeing and happiness. We feel loved and at peace with ourselves for a major part of our lives when we make this attitude ours. This adds and helps us to get rid of greed, amenity, bitterness, jealousy, and promotes a healthy and nurturing attitude towards others, which in turn gets reciprocated and we feel the sense of healthy living. We attach so much importance to this attitude of gratitude that when our children fail to thank someone, we insist that they do it. That is what is needed to be avoided from time to time. We expect this in return from others when we help them or give them a gift. We call a person discourteous and rude when they do not say thank us in return. On the face of it we ought to know that a positive is not an attitude of being satisfied and content, that you never want to do anything, anymore. This is an attitude that makes you feel good about who you are, what you do, and what your potentials are. This attitude impels you to utilize all that you are endowed with as a person, to achieve the highest possible goals. When we have this attitude, we are able to work without any external pressure to perform but there is sufficient pressure and motivation from within.The possessing of positive thinking is like any other habit, so we need to follow the routine of habit formation here as well. You will win new friends and admirers without having to impress them or conform to the pressure of doing things their way. You will be bubbling with life and the joie de vivre. You will be rearing to go and accomplish all you can with your new found confidence. The best part of adopting the 'positive thinking and a positive attitude of gratitude is that, you will be able to enjoy the smallest pleasures of nature with a heightened sense of satisfaction and awe. I can see and watch a beautiful flower and carry that joy in my mind for future enjoyment with a clear positive habit. I can go back to work freshen and can use it as an object to meditate on when I feel stressed. Let us be clear that a positive is not an attitude of being satisfied and content, that you never want to do anything, anymore. This is an attitude that makes you feel good about who you are, what you do, and what your potentials are. This attitude impels you to utilize all that you are endowed with as a person, to achieve the highest possible goals. When we have this attitude, we are able to work without any external pressure to perform but there is sufficient pressure and motivation from within. The habit of positive thinking is like any other habit, so we need to follow the routine of habit formation here as well.

HAPPINESS LIES IN POSITIVE LIVING

BE POSITVE THINK POSITIVE LIVE POSITIVE

CHAPTER FORTY SEVEN

FORGET WORRIES

Being a positive thinker is not about ignoring reality in favor of aspirational thoughts. It is more about taking a proactive approach to your life. Instead of feeling hopeless or overwhelmed, positive thinking allows you to tackle life's challenges by looking for effective ways to resolve conflict and come up with creative solutions to problems. It might not be easy, but the positive impact it will have on your mental, emotional, and physical health will be well-worth it. At time we may think that there is no road is left for us from where we can achieve the happiness of our lives. We may also feel that life has become terrible for us to live and we are carrying new hope that someone would come to rescue us. There may be chances that someone who was there with us before might have held on to us when we were on the dark side of the life. What if when everything goes wrong and all the doors of happiness are closed our live becomes a silent. It is a quite common and we are aware of a marvelous proverb that Life itself is a stage and we all are the performers, performing different acts assigned to us by our almighty power. We should not forget as to what is in our possession?, if it is to fulfill our duties towards our responsibility and do whatever is correct and is allowed by us in our life?. We should not forget that happiness in life comes through the doors of positive thoughts; we need to have them first. If one door happen to close, another opens, in the event only when we are confident and optimistic. We have so many reasons to cry and at the same time plenty of reasons to smile as well. Similarly, happiness does not stand for anything, but is on our way of thinking that how do we keep ourselves happy in life. Failure and disappointment are part of our life. The only thing is that we need to face and solve the problem is by keeping our dreams and hope alive be it a reason that success and happiness will come our way again. There are quite a number of reasons to believe that for a successful and happy life the mystery surrounding it lies in our interests, and good memory which is the basis of our interest, power of desire and aim, keeping ourselves smiling and the doubt free character which is the foremost important reason for a successful and happy life. If we possess one solid unselfish and doubt free character within ourselves we would be quite happy and successful. The experience has taught us that we should buy some strength, hope and positivity from our loved ones to help ourselves in such a situation rather than surrendering as life is a precious gift of God and is equipped with full of joy and happiness if we help ourselves in these critical moments we can live with considerable optimism. Now let's us imagine that we are not feeling at our best today, and we are having thoughts that could be classified as negative. We shouldn't be thinking such negative thoughts. We don't like the negative thoughts. We ought to know that negative thoughts are stressful, demoralizing and depressing. We shouldn't aim to have negative thoughts at all. Often we feel uncomfortable because we think we have to say or do something in response to another person's words. When we find ourselves thinking this way, it helps enormously to take a few moments to check inside and notice what we are feeling. We are deeply depressed that negativity has governed us and has taken a deep root in our minds.So, let's imagine that you have chosen to focus on your negative thinking with regards to school. The next step is to spend a little bit of time each day evaluating your own thoughts. When you find yourself thinking critical thoughts about yourself, take a moment to pause and reflect. While you might be upset about getting a bad grade on an exam, is berating yourself really the best approach? Is there any way to put a positive spin on the situation? While you might not have done well on this exam, at least you have a better indication of how to structure your study time for the next big test.

However, despite of all these good thoughts which are embodied to us by the almighty fail to revive these unwanted circumstances that lead us to sorrow and difficulties and a situation where we do not know what is correct and good for us and what is wrong for us. We should always remember that, "Life is there, where there is hope". That single thing that remains in our hands is to find out ways to know how to overcome these worries of our life at that very moment when all doors are closed for us which means that whatever situation is there, we must not give up hope. We must fight because there have been always a chance that with good faith and hard work we can turn the odds in our favor. It is often said that it is very easy to advice but when it comes to us, things go out of our control and we fail to suggest a way out for ourselves. We fall into the trap of unnecessary worries and elope ourselves with negative thoughts. We feel better when somebody else is facing some difficulty but when it comes to us we fail to gather that faith, will power and the words of strength. Being a positive thinker is not about ignoring reality in favor of aspirational thoughts.

It is more about taking a proactive approach to your life. Instead of feeling hopeless or overwhelmed, positive thinking allows you to tackle life's challenges by looking for effective ways to resolve conflict and come up with creative solutions to problems. It might not be easy, but the positive impact it will have on your mental, emotional, and physical health will be well-worth it. It takes practice; lots of practice. This is not a step-by-step process that you can complete and be done with. Instead, it involves a lifelong commitment to looking inside yourself and being willing to challenge negative thoughts and make positive changes.It is a common fact that no one in this world is free of obstacles or difficulties. If all the openings of happiness are shut for us and we have to overcome that and have no way to come out, but to survive lest we must have to learn to swim out of the sorrows because this is what is called life and sorrow free living. There are lot more examples and in many other situations, where we

will find that how we could have faced and fought with our
sorrows and difficulties of life when there was no hope left in our
lives. When the power of will is at the worst and each one of us
knows that the one who is gone never comes back. Neither a
thousands of words would not be enough to bring him back nor a
million tears, because each and every moment, eyes would only
shed tears , mind would remain tensed and we would be simply
surrounded by worries and the life seems to have been vanished.
Life is ever expanding, contraction is death. As commonly said
by big saints that the self- seeking man who is looking after his
personal comforts and leading a lazy life for himself there would
be no room for him even in the hell and he simply have lost the
power of his will. One cannot do anything without it. We fail
only when we do not try very hard to achieve the power and faith
within us. As soon as we lose faith, death comes in our way and
we are surrounds by all the evils and stupid worries of the world.
The secret and history of every successful man is to have, good
confidence, faith and strength behind him and that remain the
right cause of his single success in life. Unselfishness plays a
very vital role in his life. He may not have been perfectly
unselfish, yet he was tending towards it. If he had been perfectly
unselfish, he would have been as great a success. The degree of
unselfishness marks the degree of success everywhere and he
leads to be successful man without fear worries and selfishness.
Therefore creation of positivity in life is utmost necessary to
enjoy the special gift of God to us. The love for God and
worshipping God adds to one common thing the immense faith
in Him. There may be different beliefs and ways to worship God
in different communities, places and religions, but one thing
remains the same and that is the . Love of God for all of us. Our
world is full of odds and evens, happiness and sorrows,
fulfilment and emptiness. And these are all created by the
Almighty. However, the most beautiful Gift of God, is Human,
which is such a mystery driven by Him which could hardly be
defined or explained in depth. We know that life cannot be
foreseen. Life is not a bed of roses. Life is a battle field and not a

bed of roses as every man on earth has to struggle very hard in making his life happy. If aim of our life is to stay happy and let others to be happy, we will be happy and remembered by all. But no one will actually remember us for the wealth we have gained, or success we have achieved. I have no aim in life. Summary living with no purpose in life is just like a feather moving towards the wind. Life is such a special gift of Almighty and it is not gifted by Him to use it the way we like or love to. The actual path shown by Him needs to be followed by us for us to reach the peak of betterment every moment. We need to have some positive attitude to look at it comfortably but at the same time having a positive mental attitude does not mean banishing all negative thoughts and people from your life. One and another one arises. Change your attitude from negative thinking to Positive Thinking and converge yourself from negativity to positivity. Positive thinking is a mental and emotional attitude that focuses on the bright side of life and expects positive results. A positive person anticipates happiness, health and success, and believes he or she can overcome any obstacle and difficulty. Positive thinking is not accepted by everyone. Some, consider it as nonsense, and scoff at people who follow it, but there is a growing number of people, who accept positive thinking as a fact, and believe in its effectiveness. We need to learn a lesson from every situation. No matter how difficult the situation may appear. We should recognize the beautiful lessons waiting to be discovered. Sometimes lessons may prove to be expensive and costly, but every problem is a learning experience in disguise. We need to be conscious of our thoughts, especially, when life just isn't going our way. The moment we see that we are diving into frustration, agony, sorrow or low self –esteem we must shift our thoughts, by thinking about something completely different and unrelated.

Negative thinking is contagious.

We affect, and are affected by the people we meet, in one way or another. This happens instinctively and on a subconscious level, through words, thoughts and feelings, and through body language. Is it any wonder that we want to be around positive people, and prefer to avoid negative ones? People are more disposed to help us, if we are positive, and they dislike and avoid anyone broadcasting negativity. Negative thoughts, words and attitude, create negative and unhappy feelings, moods and behavior. When the mind is negative, poisons are released into the blood, which cause more unhappiness and negativity. This is the way to failure, frustration and disappointment. Individuals with a pessimistic explanatory style often blame themselves when bad things happen, but fail to give themselves adequate credit for successful outcomes. They also have a tendency to view negative events as expected and lasting. As you can imagine, blaming yourself for events outside of your control or viewing these unfortunate events as a persistent part of your life can have a detrimental impact on your state of mind. Positive thinkers are more apt to use an optimistic explanatory style, but the way in which people attribute events can also vary depending upon the exact situation. This will strangle the pattern of self-pity, mind-created imaginations, and negative downward stairs. Really what makes us different from other mammals is our ability to control our thoughts and think for ourselves positively and shift our negative thoughts to a positive angle. We may have made mistakes, but now we can accept it and continue, knowing that we will make a different decision in the future. If we understand this it can be appreciative for the experience. We cannot be both angry and grateful at the same time. We should start counting the blessings and miracles in our lives and if we start exploring for them and we would find more. It's quite true that we are alive and breathing! We have to realize how lucky we are with all the positivity in abundance in our lives. Our mind and body becomes dumb and mum when it comes to pressure, all it wants to do is take the easiest way out and to throw out of us our negative within us. While the terms positive thinking and positive psychology are sometimes used interchangeably, it is important to understand that they are not the same thing. First, positive thinking is about looking at things from a positive point of view. Positive psychology certainly tends to focus on optimism, but it also notes that while there are many benefits to thinking positively, there are actually times when more realistic thinking is more advantageous. Feeling good about ourselves and showing self-confidence boosts our skills potential and capabilities in any areas of work and supports us to become more positive. We need to shift our thoughts from being a negative person to more strong a positive man. Also keeping in mind that pushing things to the limit and going beyond what we think is possible for us to get to the next step of being positive. It becomes another key to achieving what we really want to do. You have probably had someone tell you to "look on the bright side" or to "see the cup as half full." Chances are good that the people who make these comments are positive thinkers. Even if it may even be relationships and we are finding it difficult to meet someone where we are actually interested in, we need not wait because it usually doesn't come to us by own, we must stand up to get help from any learned fellow. One of the most important things while doing all of this is to be happy about what we are doing, thus we ought to have a successful goal setting our lifestyle with a positive attitude.

At times we may suffer from chronic depression, though we know how good things look on to others life cannot be worse for us. Let's imagine how to deal when life leaves a great big steaming pile at our doorstep. Lest we need to remember that external factors can be dealt with by taking positive steps to repair or at least address the root of the problem as best as we can. Whatever may be the primary cause of the problem, that cause must be examined first? We may or may not be able to solve the problem, per se, but at least knowing that we are taking positive steps can help us improve our outlook. It will not be easy, of course, for us and it may be like suffering a chronic disease thus we must balance ourselves as "being positive" with an understanding that the reality is, it's going to be an ongoing battle for our own survival. Depression will undermine even the strongest of wills, need help to maintain or at least be reminded of a positive outlook. Counseling, psychotherapy, and the right combination of medication will play a crucial role in helping to keep us from sinking into that very dark place that is the essence of depression. Be patient, but don't look for miracles. It may be that we will need the help of professionals throughout our lives to maintain a generally even keel. If one could "will away" depression, there would be no need of doctors or drugs. What we can do is understand why we feel like we do, and explain to our counselors that we wish it were that easy, and that we appreciate our concern towards positivity. Shifting our thoughts enables us to the right path of our positivity and thinking in its direction of positivity can make us to lead a very happy life.

FORGET NEGATIVE THINKING

Never let life's hardships disturb you .no one can avoid problems, not even saints or sages. As with any habit, the habit of remaining positive in all situations takes practice and a commitment to yourself to take control. If you tend to think positive you stand to gain all the amenities of a happy life. Positive Thinking leads you to a happy life one must not forgot the life is what you make it, so make it a happy one!. Don't worry on things that may not happen, life is too short to worry too much. Smile and be happy. Make yourself to be positive person. Don't hold onto anything that bothers your mind. It can only hurt your health and it won't help your problems at all. The people that live the longest in this world do not hold grudges or hold or fall prey into negative feelings. Visualize your worries on a large chalkboard in your mind. Watch yourself take a big eraser and erase the problems. Every time the thoughts come back into your head, see yourself with the eraser again. Keep your slate clean and form a habit of thinking positive.We must not worry about tomorrow, for tomorrow will worry about itself. Each day has enough trouble of its own. Do not anticipate trouble, or worry about what may never happen. Keep in the sunlight. Imagine every day to be a positive day and the last of a life surrounded with hopes, The hours that come unexpectedly will be much the more grateful. The mind that is anxious about future events is miserable. Present fears are less than horrible imaginings. Positive thinking is sure to ward of every odd imagination and sure to make you a happy person. Positive thinking actually means approaching life's challenges with a positive outlook. It does not necessarily mean avoiding or ignoring the bad things; instead, it involves making the most of potentially bad situations, trying to see the best in other people, and viewing yourself and your abilities in a positive light. Positive thinking centers on such things as a belief in your abilities, a positive approach to challenges, and trying to make the most of bad situations. Bad things will happen. Sometimes you will be disappointed or hurt by the actions of others. This does not mean that the world is out to get you or that all people will let you down. Instead, positive thinkers will look at the situation realistically, search for ways that they can improve the situation, and try to learn from their experiences. Positive attitude bring good cheer, remembering that the misfortunes hardest to bear are those that never happen, focus on the positive aspects of lives, rather than on the negative setbacks. Let us not waste our lives in doubts and fears. It is not work that kills us, it is worry and the negative thinking. Work is healthy; but worry is rust upon the blade. It is not movement that destroys the machinery, but friction. We need to forget the most disturbing negative thinking in our lives and opt for the positive attitude by following the principles of positive thinking. Not only can positive thinking impact your ability to cope with stress and your immunity, it also has an impact on your overall well-being.

HAPPINESS LIES IN POSITIVE LIVING

BE POSITVE THINK POSITIVE LIVE POSITIVE

CHAPTER FORTY EIGHT

WORRIES ARE REPETITIVE THOUGHTS

Negativity and worries are repetitive thoughts associated with feelings of anxiety in anticipation of some negative future event. Worries and anxious feelings lead to disasters and make our lives unhappy. If we know that our circumstances are beyond our control or power we need to change them or revise them to our liking. We must try to put a stop-less order on our worries. We must be careful and we need not permit little things which become insects of our lives to ruin our happiness. Co-operate with the inevitable. Decide just how much anxiety a thing may be worth and refuse to give in anymore. All the happiness is not given in one go it comes slowly and slowly. We must pay special attention to remain happy and be happy. Keep ourselves happy, treat our worried thoughts as valuable signals to a sweet living good and happy living.

The utmost cause of unhappiness is your state of depression. Unhappiness is not there to motivate information gathering or problem-solving. In fact it is depression that constructs the future of unhappiness. Depression is inertia. That's the thing about depression: depression is so insidious, and it compounds daily, and it's impossible to ever see the end of it.

Keep yourself happy

Depressed people think they know themselves, but maybe they only know depression. There are no hopeless than this to get depressed create unhappiness in our minds and become unhappy all the time. Our attitude towards suffering and depression becomes very important because it can affect how we cope with suffering when it arises. Depression is nourished by a lifetime of grieved and unforgiven causes. Another factor to remain unhappy is worrying about unwanted and useless things. Worry is a misuse of the imagination. To keep yourself happy, treat your worried thoughts as most unwanted assets. These are the fundamental facts you should be familiar about worries. A huge factor to stay happy is to cater your worries around, an important relationship in your life and pay special attention sustaining positive relationships. Make your mind firm and do come to a positive decision and not allow the worries to un-ease the power your mind and soul that can cause unhappiness in you.

We must free ourselves from fruitless worry.

Once a decision is carefully reached we should get busy carrying out our decisions and should not bother about all the anxieties that are about to come. When we, or any of our colleagues or associates, are about to worry about a problem, we must write it out and think of the following questions: Instead of worrying about what people say, why not spend time trying to accomplish something they may admire. What if we just acted like everything was easy? How would your life be different if we stopped worrying about things we can't control and started focusing on the things we can? Let today be the day. We must free ourselves from fruitless worry, seize the day and take effective action on things we can change thus we would see that our lives changes for the betterment and we are on the right path of a sweet, good and happy living.

STEPS FOR HAPPY LIFE AND POSITIVE LIFE

The secret of successful and happy life lies in keeping ourselves smiling and the character which is the foremost important reason that lies within us. Do not be curious about anything, but in everything, by prayer and petition, with thanksgiving, present your requests to God. Whenever your mind is tempted to jump the fence and start to worry, say this verse aloud or to yourself. You may even have to repeat it over and over again. Am I constantly striving to see the positive in every aspect of my life?. Steps for a successful and happy life. At time we may think that there is no road is left for us from where we can achieve the happiness of our lives. We may also feel that life has become terrible for us to live and we are carrying new hope that someone would come to rescue us. There may be chances that someone who was there with us before might have held on to us when we were on the dark side of the life. We should not forget that happiness in life comes through the doors of positive thoughts; we need to have them first. If one door happen to close, another opens, in the event only when we are confident and optimistic. We have so many reasons to cry and at the same time plenty of reasons to smile as well. Similarly, happiness does not stand for anything, but is on our way of thinking that how do we keep ourselves happy in life. Failure and disappointment are part of our life. The only thing is that we need to face and solve the problem is by keeping our dreams and hope alive be it a reason that success and happiness will come our way again. The experience has taught us that we should buy some strength, hope and positivity from our loved ones to help ourselves in such a situation rather than surrendering as life is a precious gift of God.

What if when everything goes wrong and all the doors of happiness are closed our live becomes a silent. It is a quite common and we are aware of a marvelous proverb that Life itself is a stage and we all are the performers, performing different acts assigned to us by our almighty power. We should not forget as to what is in our possession if it is to fulfill our duties towards our responsibility and do whatever is correct and is allowed by us in our life?. However, despite of all these good thoughts which are embodied to us by the almighty fail to revive these unwanted circumstances that lead us to sorrow and difficulties and a situation where we do not know what is correct and good for us and what is wrong for us. We should always remember that, "Life is there, where there is hope". That single thing that remains in our hands is to find out ways to know how to overcome these worries of our life at that very moment when all doors are closed for us which means that whatever situation is there, we must not give up hope. We must fight because there have been always a chance that with good faith and hard work we can turn the odds in our favor. It is often said that it is very easy to advice but when it comes to us, things go out of our control and we fail to suggest a way out for ourselves. We fall into the trap of unnecessary worries and elope ourselves with negative thoughts. We feel better when somebody else is facing some difficulty but when it comes to us we fail to gather that faith, will power and the words of strength. It is a common fact that no one in this world is free of obstacles or difficulties. If all the openings of happiness are shut for us and we have to overcome that and have no way to come out, but to survive lest we must have to learn to swim out of the sorrows because this is what is called life and sorrow free living. There are lot more examples and in many other situations, where we will find that how we could have faced and fought with our sorrows and difficulties of life when there was no hope left in our lives. When the power of will is at the worst and each one of us knows that the one who is gone never comes back. Neither a thousands of words would not be enough to bring him back nor a million tears, because each and every moment, eyes would only shed tears , mind would remain tensed and we would be simply surrounded by worries and the life seems to have been vanished. Life is ever expanding, contraction is death. As commonly said by big saints that the self- seeking man who is looking after his personal comforts and leading a lazy life for himself there would be no room for him even in the hell and he simply have lost the power of his will.

We are quite aware of the fact that faith in oneself is the history of a man and that faith calls the quality of superiority within a person. One cannot do anything without it. We fail only when we do not try very hard to achieve the power and faith within us. As soon as we lose faith, death comes in our way and we are surrounds by all the evils and stupid worries of the world. The secret and history of every successful man is to have, good confidence, faith and strength behind him and that remain the right cause of his single success in life. Unselfishness plays a very vital role in his life. He may not have been perfectly unselfish, yet he was tending towards it. If he had been perfectly unselfish, he would have been as great a success. The degree of unselfishness marks the degree of success everywhere and he leads to be successful man without fear worries and selfishness. There are quite a number of reasons to believe that for a successful and happy life the mystery surrounding it lies in our interests, and good memory which is the basis of our interest, power of desire and aim, keeping ourselves smiling and the doubt free character which is the foremost important reason for a successful and happy life. If we possess one solid unselfish and doubt free character within ourselves we would be quite happy and successful. The love for God and worshipping God adds to one common thing the immense faith in Him. There may be different beliefs and ways to worship God in different communities, places and religions, but one thing remains the same and that is the Love of God for all of us. Our world is full of odds and evens, happiness and sorrows, fulfilment and emptiness. And these are all created by the Almighty. However, the most beautiful Gift of God, is Human, which is such a mystery driven by Him which could hardly be defined or explained in depth. We know that life cannot be foreseen. Life is not a bed of roses. Life is a battle field and not a bed of roses as every man on earth has to struggle very hard in making his life happy. If aim of our life is to stay happy and let others to be happy, we will be happy and remembered by all. But no one will actually remember us for the wealth we have gained, or success we have achieved. I have no aim in life. Summary living with no purpose in life is just like a feather moving towards the wind. Both career and purpose are different issues but it is equally important to understand the value of these things which would ultimately add spicy flavor to your living .Innovation at work place is what it necessary is how well we judge our work, how good we like and enjoy it. If we take our work as a stiff challenge and as learning everyday then we would start loving it and giving our best.

However, if we just work for the sake of then nothing is realized and we do not remain happy in life. Life is such a special gift of Almighty and it is not gifted by Him to use it the way we like or love to. The actual path shown by Him needs to be followed by us for us to reach the peak of betterment every moment. We need to have some positive attitude to look at it comfortably but at the same time having a positive mental attitude does not mean banishing all negative thoughts and people from your life. The same is true with thoughts. When we go to field with negative thoughts, we banish one and another one arises. Therefore creation of positivity in life is utmost necessary to enjoy the special gift of God to us. Now let's us imagine that we are not feeling at our best today, and we are having thoughts that could be classified as negative. We shouldn't be thinking such negative thoughts. We don't like the negative thoughts. We ought to know that negative thoughts are stressful, demoralizing and depressing. We shouldn't aim to have negative thoughts at all. Often we feel uncomfortable because we think we have to say or do something in response to another person's words. When we find ourselves thinking this way, it helps enormously to take a few moments to check inside and notice what we are feeling. We are deeply depressed that negativity has governed us and has taken a deep root in our minds. If we want to live a positive, joyful life, we must not be surrounded by negative people who don't encourage our happiness. As a negative person, we ought to get attracted too negative people only. Only when we decide to make the change to live a more positive life, we have to get rid of our lives of the most negative influences in it. We are quite aware of the fact that no one is perfect and perfection isn't the goal when it comes to positivity but there were people in our lives who were consistently negative, who constantly bring us down, we need to stop spending so much time with them. We can very well imagine, it is not easy for us to get away from these negative people. It can hurt us to keep distance from people even when you know they aren't good for us and for our current lifestyle. In addition to removing negative influences from them, we also have to get rid of some of our own negative behaviors, such as the drug and alcohol abuse. We need to take some concrete steps and examine which behaviors are good for us and which were not harmful. What we need is to learn to focus on the positive things, such as working on positive activities and cultivating new, positive relationships. We must let go of the negative ones. This process may be not easy to live a positive life when negative people and behaviors continually pull us down. In every situation or in every person there is something good. Most of the time it's not easy to find the positive qualities but we have to look hard to discover positivity in them. Now, when we are faced with a difficult or challenging situation, we need to think and talk to ourselves and console our mind, no matter how terrible the situation might seem, we can always find something good if we take the time to think about it. It is quite obvious that anything good and bad is learning experience so, at the very least, we must learn from bad experiences. However, there's usually even more to it than that. If you really take some time to have a look at it, we would find something good, something genuinely positive, about every person or situation. Once we start thinking more positively, we will realize that we had to reinforce these thoughts and behaviors within ourselves so that we could stick to it. As with any sort of training, the more we practice, the better we get to be positive. The best and easiest way to do this is to be positive when it comes to who we are. We need to speak to ourselves that we are awesome. And we have done a good job at work thus creating positivity within us. We need to be honest with ourselves, and we need to do our best to look for the good. And, whatever we do, we must not focus on the negative. It is alright not to like everything about ourselves, but don't focus on what we don't like. We have all the positive attributes, and it's up to us to remind ourselves of them every day. Not only do we need to be positive with ourselves for this multiple action to take effect, but we need to be more positive with others. We have to share our wealth of positivity with the people of the world. The best way is to be nice with other people, no matter what. Tell them that they look nice today. Appreciate their job and tell them that have done a great job on that assignment. Be positive and tell your elder or your kids how much you love them and how great they are. When someone is feeling down, do what we need to do is to cheer him or her up. Do send them gifts nice flower and glow them with nice notes.

HAPPINESS LIES IN POSITIVE LIVING
BE POSITVE THINK POSITIVE LIVE POSITIVE
CHAPTER FORTY NINE
WE MUST LEARN TO SWIM OUT OF SORROWS

It is a common fact that no one in this world is free of obstacles or difficulties. If all the openings of happiness are shut for us and we have to overcome that and have no way to come out, but to survive lest we must have to learn to swim out of the sorrows because this is what is called life and sorrow free living. There are lot more examples and in many other situations, where we will find that how we could have faced and fought with our sorrows and difficulties of life when there was no hope left in our lives.

Fighting for survival is what is needed at odd intervals.

Once we start thinking more positively and happily, we will realize that we had to reinforce these thoughts and behaviors within ourselves so that we could stick to it. As with any sort of training, the more we practice, the better we get to be positive. The best and easiest way to do this is to be positive when it comes to who we are. We need to speak to ourselves that we are awesome. And we have done a good job at work thus creating positivity within us. We need to be honest with ourselves, and we need to do our best to look for the good. And, whatever we do, we must not focus on the negative but focus as to how we can become happy by discarding all negative thoughts and have the feeling to remain happy and gay. It is alright not to like everything about ourselves, but don't focus on what we don't like. We have all the positive attributes, and it's up to us to remind ourselves of them every day in order to make us to live happily in our lives.

Life is such a special gift of Almighty so always be happy

Life is such a special gift of Almighty and it is not gifted by Him to use it the way we like or love to. The actual path shown by Him needs to be followed by us for us to reach the peak of betterment every moment. We need to have some happy attitude to look at it comfortably but at the same time having a positive mental attitude does not mean banishing all negative thoughts and people from your life. The same is true with thoughts. When we go to field with negative thoughts, we banish one and another one arises. Therefore creation of positivity and creation of happiness in life is utmost necessary to enjoy the special gift of God to us.

Do not create unnecessary worries.

If we try to change the way we look, talk and behave just to please others, and show our pride we will gradually become such a person that we ourselves won't recognize each other and would start and create unnecessary worries within us and our surrounding without being positive and will not start to live happily. Thus we must behave in such a manner so as not to create unnecessary worries in our thoughts and mind. We ought to stop worrying over unnecessary things be positive and live without fear happily. We need to understand that what people think of us is their concern, and not ours.

If they think about us to be, too reticent or proud, it's really not our business. If every time we happen to meet some new fellows, we may wonder and imagine as what they think of us, and with this feeling in us we will never be able to live a trouble-free and hassle free life. We are bound to fall into the trap of unnecessary worries denying us the startup of new and the happy living life. We would not be able to lead a sweet good and happy life. The main reason is that we must think rationally. Is it in our hands or can we control what others think about us? Simply we need to ignore them. If we cannot, and live our lives the way we want to and find the ways to leave worries aside and start living a happy life. Let us make our way to happy living.

Happy Living with Positive Attitudes.

Positive thinking is not about putting on a pair of rose-colored glasses and ignoring all the negative things you will encounter in life. That approach can be just as devastating as ignoring the positive and only focusing on the negative. Balance, with a healthy dose of realism, is the key. It is a well-known fact that attitude decides how a natives or persons copes up with the day to day events of life. Attitude is what a influence a person's reaction to a situation in life is. It sets the emotional undertone for a person to his likes or dislikes a situation even before he is acquainted with it. Positive attitude is a quality that is second to none in a human being. Though we attach so much importance to this attitude, as we grow into teenage and adult years we find ourselves becoming ungrateful or taking things for granted. We lose touch with the very same qualities that we instill in our children. We take for granted our life, our health, our families, the people in our lives, the things that our loved ones do for us to make our lives easier and things that we possess.

The positive attitude and happy face speaks a lot about a person.

It denotes about changing negative happiness and making positive thinking and living a positive attitude a good habit. Thinking positively and a positive attitude help us to appreciate and value ourselves, our potential and all that we have. It ensures that we do not take our abilities for granted. It makes us look at ourselves as special people with a special set of abilities and potential. It banishes the feelings of inadequacy and insecurity that arises from unfair comparisons with others. It helps us to appreciate people for who they are and not magnify what they are not and their little flaws. It drives away prejudice and makes us approach life with an open mind. It predisposes us to react to the daily events of life in a positive manner and help us to look at the brighter side of life. Make us optimistic. It gives hope and helps us look forward to life with anticipation and makes us to live happily. We need to know that positive thinking takes the focus away from what we don't have, to appreciating and making good use of what we have. It is closely connected to our emotional wellbeing and happiness. We feel loved and at peace with ourselves for a major part of our lives when we make this attitude ours. This adds and helps us to get rid of greed, amenity, bitterness, jealousy, and promotes a healthy and nurturing attitude towards others, which in turn gets reciprocated and we feel the sense of healthy living. We attach so much importance to this attitude of gratitude that when our children fail to thank someone, we insist that they do it. That is what is needed to be avoided from time to time. We expect this in return from others when we help them or give them a gift. We call a person discourteous and rude when they do not say thank us in return. On the face of it we ought to know that a positive is not an attitude of being satisfied and content, that you never want to do anything, anymore. This is an attitude that makes you feel good about who you are, what you do, and what your potentials are. This attitude impels you to utilize all that you are endowed with as a person, to achieve the highest possible goals. When we have this attitude, we are able to work without any external pressure to perform but there is sufficient pressure and motivation from within.

The possessing of happy living is like any other habit.

The possessing of happy living is like any other habit, so you need to follow the routine of habit formation here as well. You will win new friends and admirers without having to impress them or conform to the pressure of doing things their way. You will be bubbling with life. You will be rearing to go and accomplish all you can with your new found confidence. The best part of adopting the 'happy living" is a positive attitude of gratitude is that, you will be able to enjoy the smallest pleasures of nature with a heightened sense of satisfaction and awe. You can see and watch a beautiful flower and carry that joy in your mind for future enjoyment with a clear positive habit. You can go back to work freshen and can use it as an object to meditate on when you feel stressed. You can converge to form of happy living with this habit of positive and sweet living. You need to remember that the possession of happy living is like any other habit and one need not practice so hard to get it.Let us be clear that a positive is not an attitude of being satisfied and content, that we never want to do anything, anymore. This is an attitude that makes you feel good about who you are, what you do, and what your potentials are. This attitude impels you to utilize all that you are endowed with as a person, to achieve the highest possible goals. When we have this attitude, we are able to work without any external pressure to perform but there is sufficient pressure and motivation from within. The habit of happy living is like any other habit, so we need to follow the routine of habit formation here as well.

Keeping our dreams and hope alive our success and happiness.

We should not forget that happiness in life comes through the doors of positive thoughts; we need to have them first. If one door happen to close, another opens, in the event only when we are confident and optimistic. We have so many reasons to cry and at the same time plenty of reasons to smile as well. Similarly, happiness does not stand for anything, but is on our way of thinking that how do we keep ourselves happy in life. Failure and disappointment are part of our life. The only thing is that we need to face and solve the problem is by keeping our dreams and hope alive be it a reason that success and happiness will come our way again. The experience has taught us that we should buy some strength, hope and positivity from our loved ones to help ourselves in such a situation rather than surrendering as life is a precious gift of God and is equipped with full of joy and happiness if we help ourselves in these critical moments we can live with considerable optimism.

Life is there, where there is hope.

What if when everything goes wrong and all the doors of happiness are closed our live becomes a silent. It is a quite common and we are aware of a marvelous proverb that Life itself is a stage and we all are the performers, performing different acts assigned to us by our almighty power. We should always remember that, "Life is there, where there is hope". That single thing that remains in our hands is to find out ways to know how to overcome these worries of our life at that very moment when all doors are closed for us which means that whatever situation is there, we must not give up hope. We must fight because there have been always a chance that with good faith and hard work we can turn the odds in our favor. It is often said that it is very easy to advice but when it comes to us, things go out of our control and we fail to suggest a way out for ourselves. We fall into the trap of unnecessary worries and elope ourselves with negative thoughts. We feel better when somebody else is facing some difficulty but when it comes to us we fail to gather that faith, will power and the words of strength. When the power of will is at the worst and each one of us knows that the one who is gone never comes back. Neither a thousands of words would not be enough to bring him back nor a million tears, because each and every moment, eyes would only shed tears , mind would remain tensed and we would be simply surrounded by worries and the life seems to have been vanished. Life is ever expanding, contraction is death. As commonly said by big saints that the self- seeking man who is looking after his personal comforts and leading a lazy life for himself there would be no room for him even in the hell and he simply have lost the power of his will. We are quite aware of the fact that faith in oneself is the history of a man and that faith calls the quality of superiority within a person. One cannot do anything without it. We fail only when we do not try very hard to achieve the power and faith within us. As soon as we lose faith, death comes in our way and we are surrounds by all the evils and stupid worries of the world. The secret and history of every successful man is to have, good confidence, faith and strength behind him and that remain the right cause of his single success in life. Unselfishness plays a very vital role in his life. He may not have been perfectly unselfish, yet he was tending towards it. If he had been perfectly unselfish, he would have been as great a success. The degree of unselfishness marks the degree of success everywhere and he leads to be successful man without fear worries and selfishness. There are quite a number of reasons to believe that for a successful and happy life the mystery surrounding it lies in our interests, and good memory which is the basis of our interest, power of desire and aim, keeping ourselves smiling and the doubt free character which is the foremost important reason for a successful and happy life.

The love for God and worshipping.

The love for God and worshipping God adds to one common thing the immense faith in Him. There may be different beliefs and ways to worship God in different communities, places and religions, but one thing remains the same and that is the Love of God for all of us. Our world is full of odds and evens, happiness and sorrows, fulfilment and emptiness. And these are all created by the Almighty. However, the most beautiful Gift of God, is a Human, which is such a mystery driven by Him which could hardly be defined or explained in depth.

The secret of successful and happy life lies in keeping ourselves smiling.

The secret of successful and happy life lies in keeping ourselves smiling and the character which is the foremost important reason that lies within us. Do not be curious about anything, but in everything, by prayer and petition, with thanksgiving, present your requests to God. Whenever your mind is tempted to jump the fence and start to worry, say this verse aloud or to yourself. You may even have to repeat it over and over again.

Steps for a successful and happy life.

Being a positive thinker is not about ignoring reality in favor of aspirational thoughts. It is more about taking a proactive approach to your life. Instead of feeling hopeless or overwhelmed, positive thinking allows you to tackle life's challenges by looking for effective ways to resolve conflict and come up with creative solutions to problems.

HAPPINESS LIES IN POSITIVE LIVING
BE POSITVE THINK POSITIVE LIVE POSITIVE
CHAPTER FIFTY
LIFE IS NOT BED OF ROSES

Life is a battle field and not a bed of roses as every man on earth has to struggle very hard in making his life happy. If aim of our life is to stay happy and let others to be happy, we will be happy and remembered by all. But no one will actually remember us for the wealth we have gained, or success we have achieved. If we have no aim in life, we would not be able to lead and happy life. Living with no purpose in life is just like a feather moving towards the wind. Both career and purpose are different issues but it is equally important to understand the value of these things which would ultimately add spicy flavor to your living. Innovation at work place is what is it necessary how well we judge our work, how good we like and enjoy it. If we take our work as a stiff challenge and as learning everyday then we would start loving it and giving our best. However, if we just work for the sake of then nothing is realized and we do not remain happy in life.

We should not aim to have negative thoughts at all.

Now let's us imagine that we are not feeling at our best today, and we are having thoughts that could be classified as negative. We shouldn't be thinking such negative thoughts. We don't like the negative thoughts. We ought to know that negative thoughts are stressful, demoralizing and depressing. We shouldn't aim to have negative thoughts at all. Often we feel uncomfortable because we think we have to say or do something in response to another person's words. When we find ourselves thinking this way, it helps enormously to take a few moments to check inside and notice what we are feeling. Negative thoughts destroy our happy livings. We ought to discard all these negative thought and act to live in a more positive atmosphere rather than living in a negative world where we can never find a happy living.

Positivity is state of mind

Positivity is something you cannot earn or buy. If you have spent your life trying to get some happiness or something that will make you happy, odds are that you are wasting a really good life that you don't know you have. You passed up and overlooked a lot of personal happiness. You are probably spending so much time chasing and dreaming of unnecessary thing of what could be of no use to you and that you are forgetting about all the small and big things occurring right now that could make you happy. People and things alone, won't make you happy. Your own efforts not to get worried or depressed make you happy. You know the saying, that "Positivity is a state of mind". And state of mind is what you think do and act in a peaceful manner without being getting worried or depressed. The best thing about happiness is that you get it is free. You don't have to pay or you do not have to open any account to be happy. You don't have to pay monthly rent for it either. You just have to change your perspective, your views on what you are seeing and feeling. Happiness is not something which is quite readymade. It comes from your own actions and deeds. Don't let one cloud darken the whole sky. Angriness and happiness don't mix. You must dig out the angriness in you, and see that the happiness has shown and seeded a place to grow its roots. The ultimate goal of life should be to get happiness and not get involved into unnecessary worries falling in the death trap of defeats and failures. The essence of life is not in the great victories and grand failures, but in the simple joys. The purpose of our lives is to be happy. Laugh when you can, apologize when you should, and let go of what you can't change. Think positive and just visualize that what is stored in destiny would not be negative. If you want to be happy, be positive first practice meditation. If you want, others to be happy practice compassion. Whoever is happy will make others happy, too.

Let us be very sure and let us keep in mind that happiness doesn't depend on any superficial conditions, it is governed by our mental attitude only. Our greatest gift to others is to be happy and to radiate our happiness to the entire world. Happiness is a guide to direction, not a place to hide. As a happy person, you radiate happiness to the world. Visualize your light radiating throughout the world, passing from person to person until it encircles the globe. Resolve to keep happy, and your joy and you shall form an invincible host against difficulties. The positive persons often dance to the happy tunes of their lives. The path to happiness is forgiveness of everyone and gratitude for everything. Happiness fills your heart each day and your whole life through with clean thoughts. Any day would be a wonderful day if you do not to take life so seriously. Happiness is not about being a winner -it's about being gentle with life being gentle within you. Happiness blooms in the presence of self-respect and the absence of ego. Love yourself. Love everyone around you. Love everyone in the whole world. When you're feeling depressed or anxious, close your eyes and try to visualize a guided positive imaginary thing. First breathe deeply and relax. How important it is to consistently reach for positive, uplifting, inspirational thoughts. Thought that promote aliveness and abundance. Thoughts that make you feel good. Look at the birds of the air; they do not sow or reap or store away in barns, and yet our heavenly Father feeds them. Imagine that you're already a positive person and you love life. The only thing between us and our desire, to be happy, is one single fact: we are not happy because we often fall into the death trap of depression and wholly because of our negative thoughts. Absence of positive thinking, has eluded us of our great happiness and left us far behind. This very little known fact has kept many of us from reaching our goal of happiness. If you keep thinking things like as if your life is dead!", nothing would be achieved and it will be like that only. Throw away all your negative thoughts and worries, concentrate on the goals to be achieved, on the ray of happiness in you and make sure that you are not falling again into the path of negativity. "Happiness is a state of mind only and not the thoughts of negatives, and it quite true that happiness can only be achieved if you have a positive mind and a clear attitude of being a positive person. Happiness and positivity go hand in hand. If you are positive you are a happy person and if you possess negativity you would land yourself to be a very negative person thus ruining your life for what of nothing.

Have Positive Thinking

Have Positive Thinking, think positive as all your thoughts, good and bad, are the creation of your mind which tends to lead you to a materialistic life and go in to generate unnecessary worries. Thus you will learn to be more positive. The environment and all the experiences in your life are the results of your habitual and dominant thoughts. Positive thoughts bring good and happiness. Negative thoughts could tell us about something that needs special attention when they lead us to the path of worries. We must discover what needs to be done, and think positively to take care of it. Many of us fail to see a negative occurrence and do not think of a replacement of negative thought with positive one. As they even do not even dare look for a bright side in every situation. If we do this for a longer period of time, we become habitual, and it will make a tremendous delay in improving our positive thinking skills. We must remember, everything can be framed positively if we make a restless effort to do so. Positive thinking wards off the ingredients of negative thoughts in our minds there are both positive and negative aspects to most situations. We get to choose which ones we will focus on. We can try to catch ourselves when we're being negative and do not try thinking the positive side of the things. There's no sense in worrying about the negatives if these negatives cannot be changed. If we waste energy and happiness on the things we can't change, we'll only make ourselves more frustrated and come to the stage of depression dejection and disappointments. Negativity is a habit and we often don't realize we're doing ourselves down. Under each negative thought that we have written, we can spot an alternative way of looking at it, that isn't so negative. Take your mind to positivity and mold and drive your thoughts to the positivity. There's a world of difference between expecting failure or rejection so as not to be disappointed when it occurs and recognizing it as a possibility of being positive. It's sensible to look at a situation from all angles and to have a back-up plan to fall back on if need be. People who do this will not see failure as another step on the road to eventual success; but by expecting and envisioning success, there's less likely to be a failure. Let us find some ways of removing negative thoughts and discouraging our worries to be born.

The first step is by way of giving a good smile.

The easiest way is smiling. Many theories have revealed that even a forced smile can lift one's mood and can divert your mind to positive thinking.. We may also share positivity with others by flashing them with a brilliant and good smile. Positive Thinking is a reward of good Smiling and not a risk. The only thing we risk when we think positive is giving ourselves a little more happiness.

The second good step is to have the company of positive thinking friends.

Keep yourself busy and surround yourself with good friends, who always think positive. Appreciate the people in your life who have stood by you through thick and thin. Count their support and analyses the positivity in them which will help you to become more positive, and in the process you will probably help them too. Good friends help each other in the days of crises and through both the good and bad times. Feel positive about them and feel lucky to have them in your company. Share positive thoughts with them. Tell them to be more positive in live.

The third step is to focus your imagination on positive thoughts

Focus your imagination and make efforts on becoming new positive person. Create positivizes in you. Divert your mind to positive thinking. It is much easier to bring about change if you just put your mind to it and change your thoughts into a much more positive direction. We know that it is difficult for us to control things that happen in our lives, but we can, with some effort, control what we think or do in our lives. Positive thinking will make our imagination livelier and we would be able to lead our lives without many worries. Dejection, Disappointments and Depression, however, has consequences that could ruin our, health, and well-being. This is the reason why many people suffer from depression much more often in winter than in the other seasons. It's because the days are shorter and do not divert their minds to focus to the imagination of positive thinking.

HAPPINESS LIES IN POSITIVE LIVING
BE POSITVE THINK POSITIVE LIVE POSITIVE
CHAPTER FIFTY ONE
LIFE IS TO LIVE HAPPILY

Annalise sweet good and happy living and stop worrying over petty matters. Generate sweet living and generate good thoughts. Don't wait around or expect others to create happiness that is entirely yours to make. Whatever your goal is, do whatever you have to do to get it, always keep yourself to be a happy person. Why worry about the future. Just imagine as to what if we just acted like everything was easy and there was nothing very serious about it to come in future. Worry often gives a small thing a big shadow and its surrounding do frightened with more scary things with the result we do not tend to have a happy life or a sweet and happing living.

Make yourself aware of what's possible in this world.

Worrying will carry tomorrow's load with today's strength. Worry will not empty tomorrow of its sorrows, but it tends to empty today of its power and strength. Worries make you to move into tomorrow ahead of time. Half the worry in the world is caused by people trying to make decisions before they have sufficient knowledge on which to base a decision. Their negative thoughts pressurise them to be away from the positivity in their lives as they fail and do not analysis on positive and they fail to lead a happy life or sweet life.

Why worry about tomorrow;

Concentrate on today happening as for tomorrow will worry about itself. Each day has its own worries and troubles. Always think that you are a happy man. If there is not any solution to the some problem then do not waste time worrying about it. And if there is a solution to the problem then why waste time worrying about it. Act fast be happy generate positive happiness worries will automatically vanish in the air and you are sure to lead a sweet life and happy life.

The first step to good and happy is by way of creating good and happy thoughts in your minds.

Focus your imagination and make efforts on becoming new positive person. Create happiness in you. Divert your mind to good thoughts. It is much easier to bring about change if you just put your mind to it and change your thoughts into a much more positive direction. We know that it is difficult for us to control things that happen in our lives, but we can, with some effort, control what we think or do in our lives. Positive thoughts will make our imagination livelier and we would be able to lead our lives happily without many worries.

The second good step is to have the company of good and positive living friends.

Appreciate the people in your life who have stood by you through thick and thin. Count their support and analyses the happiness in them which will help you to lead a much happier life. Good friends help each other in the days of crises and through both the good and bad times. Keep yourself busy and surround yourself with good friends, who always think positive. Feel positive about them and feel lucky to have them in your company. Share positive thoughts with them. Tell them to be happy and to lead a sweet good and happy life.

The third step is to focus your imagination on happy things in life by giving a good smile.

The easiest way is feeling happy. Many theories have revealed that happiness can lift one's mood and can divert your mind to sweet living. We may also share positivity with others by flashing them with a brilliant and good smile. Positive and sweet talks are the rewards of good and happy thoughts it generates more happiness. Dejection, disappointments and depression, however, have consequences that could ruin our health, and life. We must divert their minds to focus to the imagination of good and happy life. If something bad or good is to happen it is sure to happen, whether we are sad or unhappy or depressed. Let us put our energy into today and stop worrying about the future and past. We should not foresee trouble, or worry about what may never happen as past is dead and gone forever and future is uncertain and yet to come. Be your unabashed self in all the best ways that you can.

The basic facts we should know about happiness.

The basic techniques to analyze happiness and how to break the unhappy habits before it breaks us. These are the simple ways where we can concentrate and get rid of unhappy thoughts. Annalise unhappiness to see and get the reasons and facts as to why we worry. To avoid reoccurrence of worries, concentrate on prayers as prayers are the best source of remedies of the prevailing worries. The more you pray, the less you'll panic. The more you worship, the less you worry. There is nothing that wastes the body like worry, and anyone who has any faith in God should need not to worry about anything whatsoever is to happen in future. This will ease our way to a sweet good and happy living.

What do we think about happy thoughts?

The feeling of happiness   is within us. It is said that sweet good and happy living is purely our own matter and it has nothing to do with our external circumstances. There is something very special within us which keeps us happy and there is something very unpleasant within us which keeps unhappy. Yes quite true it is the positivizes within us that make and creates happiness within us .Happy living through positivity is nothing more than that of living a normal life free from undue pressures, problems and tensions. If we want to live a happy life then we need to get rid of the negativity and we must try to avoid all the unpleasant things within us which makes us unhappy.

Negative approach always complicates the problems and increases unhappiness.

Most of us do the fatal mistake of looking outwards for happiness rather than looking inwards. Be happy, be strong, be bold and be courageous every day. Even if we are having a bad day, think of some good things that may come our way, either later that day, tomorrow, next week, month, or next moment.

Simply making castles in the air won't solve our problems.

When everything seems to be beyond our control, it's almost too easy for us to slip into the grasp of unhappiness. To avoid unhappiness we must strive to abolish this sort of thinking through the power of thinking positively. We ought to know the basic fundamental of analyzing happiness. Worries and unhappiness create unnecessary thoughts and these are caused by people going in for unwanted decisions, fore hand not even knowing as to when a good decision is made and not even having sufficient knowledge about it. We must first study and after carefully weighing all the facts than only come to a powerful decision. Simply making castles in the air won't solve our problems but add more to our vows and unhappiness which may even lead us to unhappy life. Anxiety and worry can go hand in hand. When anxiety grabs the mind, it is self-perpetuating. Your mind gets clogged with numerous buts and ifs. Do not worry about your life.

Negativity and worries are repetitive thoughts

Negativity and worries are repetitive thoughts associated with feelings of anxiety in anticipation of some negative future event. Worries and anxious feelings lead to disasters and make our lives unhappy. If we know that our circumstances are beyond our control or power we need to change them or revise them to our liking. We must try to put a stop-less order on our worries. We must be careful and we need not permit little things which become insects of our lives to ruin our happiness. Co-operate with the inevitable. Decide just how much anxiety a thing may be worth and refuse to give in anymore. All the happiness is not given in one go it comes slowly and slowly. We must pay special attention to remain happy and be happy. Keep ourselves happy, treat our worried thoughts as valuable signals to a sweet living good and happy living.**The utmost cause of unhappiness is your state of depression**. Unhappiness is not there to motivate information gathering or problem-solving. In fact it is depression that constructs the future of unhappiness. Depression is inertia.

That's the thing about depression: depression is so insidious, and it compounds daily, and it's impossible to ever see the end of it.

Keep yourself happy

Depressed people think they know themselves, but maybe they only know depression. There are no hopeless than this to get depressed create unhappiness in our minds and become unhappy all the time. Our attitude towards suffering and depression becomes very important because it can affect how we cope with suffering when it arises. Depression is nourished by a lifetime of grieved and unforgiven causes. Another factor to remain unhappy is worrying about unwanted and useless things. Worry is a misuse of the imagination. To keep yourself happy, treat your worried thoughts as most unwanted assets. These are the fundamental facts you should be familiar about worries. A huge factor to stay happy is to cater your worries around, an important relationship in your life and pay special attention sustaining positive relationships. Make your mind firm and do come to a positive decision and not allow the worries to un-ease the power your mind and soul that can cause unhappiness in you.

We must free ourselves from fruitless worry.

Once a decision is carefully reached we should get busy carrying out our decisions and should not bother about all the anxieties that are about to come. When we, or any of our colleagues or associates, are about to worry about a problem, we must write it out and think of the following questions: Instead of worrying about what people say, why not spend time trying to accomplish something they may admire. What if we just acted like everything was easy? How would your life be different if we stopped worrying about things we can't control and started focusing on the things we can? Let today be the day. We must free ourselves from fruitless worry, seize the day and take effective action on things we can change thus we would see that our lives changes for the betterment and we are on the right path of a sweet, good and happy living.

HAPPINESS LIES IN POSITIVE LIVING
BE POSITVE THINK POSITIVE LIVE POSITIVE
CHAPTER FIFTY TWO
WHY WORRY AND UNHAPPY LIVING

It is a common fact that no one in this world is free of obstacles or difficulties. If all the openings of happiness are shut for us and we have to overcome that and have no way to come out, but to survive lest we must have to learn to swim out of the sorrows because this is what is called life and sorrow free living. There are lot more examples and in many other situations, where we will find that how we could have faced and fought with our sorrows and difficulties of life when there was no hope left in our lives.

Fighting for survival is what is needed at odd intervals.

Once we start thinking more positively and happily, we will realize that we had to reinforce these thoughts and behaviors within ourselves so that we could stick to it. As with any sort of training, the more we practice, the better we get to be positive. The best and easiest way to do this is to be positive when it comes to who we are. We need to speak to ourselves that we are awesome. And we have done a good job at work thus creating positivity within us. We need to be honest with ourselves, and we need to do our best to look for the good. And, whatever we do, we must not focus on the negative but focus as to how we can become happy by discarding all negative thoughts and have the feeling to remain happy and gay. It is alright not to like everything about ourselves, but don't focus on what we don't like. We have all the positive attributes, and it's up to us to remind ourselves of them every day in order to make us to live happily in our lives.

Life is such a special gift of Almighty so always be happy

Life is such a special gift of Almighty and it is not gifted by Him to use it the way we like or love to. The actual path shown by Him needs to be followed by us for us to reach the peak of betterment every moment. We need to have some happy attitude to look at it comfortably but at the same time having a positive mental attitude does not mean banishing all negative thoughts and people from your life. The same is true with thoughts. When we go to field with negative thoughts, we banish one and another one arises. Therefore creation of positivity and creation of happiness in life is utmost necessary to enjoy the special gift of God to us.

Do not create unnecessary worries.

If we try to change the way we look, talk and behave just to please others, and show our pride we will gradually become such a person that we ourselves won't recognize each other and would start and create unnecessary worries within us and our surrounding without being positive and will not start to live happily. Thus we must behave in such a manner so as not to create unnecessary worries in our thoughts and mind. We ought to stop worrying over unnecessary things be positive and live without fear happily. We need to understand that what people think of us is their concern, and not ours. If they think about us to be, too reticent or proud, it's really not our business. If every time we happen to meet some new fellows, we may wonder and imagine as what they think of us, and with this feeling in us we will never be able to live a trouble-free and hassle free life. We are bound to fall into the trap of unnecessary worries denying us the startup of new and the happy living life. We would not be able to lead a sweet good and happy life. The main reason is that we must think rationally. Is it in our hands or can we control what others think about us? Simply we need to ignore them. If we cannot, and live our lives the way we want to and find the ways to leave worries aside and start living a happy life. Let us make our way to happy living.

Happy Living with Positive Attitudes.

Positive thinking is not about putting on a pair of rose-colored glasses and ignoring all the negative things you will encounter in life. That approach can be just as devastating as ignoring the positive and only focusing on the negative. Balance, with a healthy dose of realism, is the key. It is a well-known fact that attitude decides how a natives or persons copes up with the day to day events of life. Attitude is what a influence a person's reaction to a situation in life is. It sets the emotional undertone for a person to his likes or dislikes a situation even before he is acquainted with it. Positive attitude is a quality that is second to none in a human being. Though we attach so much importance to this attitude, as we grow into teenage and adult years we find ourselves becoming ungrateful or taking things for granted. We lose touch with the very same qualities that we instill in our children. We take for granted our life, our health, our families, the people in our lives, the things that our loved ones do for us to make our lives easier and things that we possess.

The positive attitude and happy face speaks a lot about a person.

It denotes about changing negative happiness and making positive thinking and living a positive attitude a good habit. Thinking positively and a positive attitude help us to appreciate and value ourselves, our potential and all that we have. It ensures that we do not take our abilities for granted. It makes us look at ourselves as special people with a special set of abilities and potential. It banishes the feelings of inadequacy and insecurity that arises from unfair comparisons with others. It helps us to appreciate people for who they are and not magnify what they are not and their little flaws. It drives away prejudice and makes us approach life with an open mind. It predisposes us to react to the daily events of life in a positive manner and help us to look at the brighter side of life. Make us optimistic. It gives hope and helps us look forward to life with anticipation and makes us to live happily. We need to know that positive thinking takes the focus away from what we don't have, to appreciating and making good use of what we have. It is closely connected to our emotional wellbeing and happiness. We feel loved and at peace with ourselves for a major part of our lives when we make this attitude ours. This adds and helps us to get rid of greed, amenity, bitterness, jealousy, and promotes a healthy and nurturing attitude towards others, which in turn gets reciprocated and we feel the sense of healthy living. We attach so much importance to this attitude of gratitude that when our children fail to thank someone, we insist that they do it. That is what is needed to be avoided from time to time. We expect this in return from others when we help them or give them a gift. We call a person discourteous and rude when they do not say thank us in return.On the face of it we ought to know that a positive is not an attitude of being satisfied and content, that you never want to do anything, anymore. This is an attitude that makes you feel good about who you are, what you do, and what your potentials are. This attitude impels you to utilize all that you are endowed with as a person, to achieve the highest possible goals. When we have this attitude, we are able to work without any external pressure to perform but there is sufficient pressure and motivation from within.

The possessing of happy living is like any other habit.

The possessing of happy living is like any other habit, so you need to follow the routine of habit formation here as well. You will win new friends and admirers without having to impress them or conform to the pressure of doing things their way. You will be bubbling with life. You will be rearing to go and accomplish all you can with your new found confidence. The best part of adopting the 'happy living" is a positive attitude of gratitude is that, you will be able to enjoy the smallest pleasures of nature with a heightened sense of satisfaction and awe. You can see and watch a beautiful flower and carry that joy in your mind for future enjoyment with a clear positive habit. You can go back to work freshen and can use it as an object to meditate on when you feel stressed. You can converge to form of happy living with this habit of positive and sweet living. You need to remember that the possession of happy living is like any other habit and one need not practice so hard to get it. Let us be clear that a positive is not an attitude of being satisfied and content, that we never want to do anything, anymore. This is an attitude that makes you feel good about who you are, what you do, and what your potentials are. This attitude impels you to utilize all that you are endowed with as a person, to achieve the highest possible goals. When we have this attitude, we are able to work without any external pressure to perform but there is sufficient pressure and motivation from within. The habit of happy living is like any other habit, so we need to follow the routine of habit formation here as well.

Keeping our dreams and hope alive our success and happiness.

We should not forget that happiness in life comes through the doors of positive thoughts; we need to have them first. If one door happen to close, another opens, in the event only when we are confident and optimistic. We have so many reasons to cry and at the same time plenty of reasons to smile as well. Similarly, happiness does not stand for anything, but is on our way of thinking that how do we keep ourselves happy in life. Failure and disappointment are part of our life. The only thing is that we need to face and solve the problem is by keeping our dreams and hope alive be it a reason that success and happiness will come our way again. The experience has taught us that we should buy some strength, hope and positivity from our loved ones to help ourselves in such a situation rather than surrendering as life is a precious gift of God and is equipped with full of joy and happiness if we help ourselves in these critical moments we can live with considerable optimism.

Life is there, where there is hope.

What if when everything goes wrong and all the doors of happiness are closed our live becomes a silent. It is a quite common and we are aware of a marvelous proverb that Life itself is a stage and we all are the performers, performing different acts assigned to us by our almighty power. We should always remember that, "Life is there, where there is hope". That single thing that remains in our hands is to find out ways to know how to overcome these worries of our life at that very moment when all doors are closed for us which means that whatever situation is there, we must not give up hope. We must fight because there have been always a chance that with good faith and hard work we can turn the odds in our favor. It is often said that it is very easy to advice but when it comes to us, things go out of our control and we fail to suggest a way out for ourselves. We fall into the trap of unnecessary worries and elope ourselves with negative thoughts. We feel better when somebody else is facing some difficulty but when it comes to us we fail to gather that faith, will power and the words of strength. When the power of will is at the worst and each one of us knows that the one who is gone never comes back. Neither a thousands of words would not be enough to bring him back nor a million tears, because each and every moment, eyes would only shed tears , mind would remain tensed and we would be simply surrounded by worries and the life seems to have been vanished. Life is ever expanding, contraction is death. As commonly said by big saints that the self- seeking man who is looking after his personal comforts and leading a lazy life for himself there would be no room for him even in the hell and he simply have lost the power of his will.We are quite aware of the fact that faith in oneself is the history of a man and that faith calls the quality of superiority within a person. One cannot do anything without it. We fail only when we do not try very hard to achieve the power and faith within us. As soon as we lose faith, death comes in our way and we are surrounds by all the evils and stupid worries of the world.The secret and history of every successful man is to have, good confidence, faith and strength behind him and that remain the right cause of his single success in life. Unselfishness plays a very vital role in his life. He may not have been perfectly unselfish, yet he was tending towards it. If he had been perfectly unselfish, he would have been as great a success. The degree of unselfishness marks the degree of success everywhere and he leads to be successful man without fear worries and selfishness. There are quite a number of reasons to believe that for a successful and happy life the mystery surrounding it lies in our interests, and good memory which is the basis of our interest, power of desire and aim, keeping ourselves smiling and the doubt free character which is the foremost important reason for a successful and happy life.

The love for God and worshipping.

The love for God and worshipping God adds to one common thing the immense faith in Him. There may be different beliefs and ways to worship God in different communities, places and religions, but one thing remains the same and that is the Love of God for all of us. Our world is full of odds and evens, happiness and sorrows, fulfilment and emptiness. And these are all created by the Almighty. However, the most beautiful Gift of God, is a Human, which is such a mystery driven by Him which could hardly be defined or explained in depth.

The secret of successful and happy life lies in keeping ourselves smiling.

The secret of successful and happy life lies in keeping ourselves smiling and the character which is the foremost important reason that lies within us. Do not be curious about anything, but in everything, by prayer and petition, with thanksgiving, present your requests to God. Whenever your mind is tempted to jump the fence and start to worry, say this verse aloud or to yourself. You may even have to repeat it over and over again.

Steps for a successful and happy life.

Being a positive thinker is not about ignoring reality in favor of aspirational thoughts. It is more about taking a proactive approach to your life. Instead of feeling hopeless or overwhelmed, positive thinking allows you to tackle life's challenges by looking for effective ways to resolve conflict and come up with creative solutions to problems.

Life is not a bed of roses.

Life is a battle field and not a bed of roses as every man on earth has to struggle very hard in making his life happy. If aim of our life is to stay happy and let others to be happy, we will be happy and remembered by all. But no one will actually remember us for the wealth we have gained, or success we have achieved. If we have no aim in life, we would not be able to lead and happy life. Living with no purpose in life is just like a feather moving towards the wind. Both career and purpose are different issues but it is equally important to understand the value of these things which would ultimately add spicy flavor to your living.Innovation at work place is what it necessary is how well we judge our work, how good we like and enjoy it. If we take our work as a stiff challenge and as learning everyday then we would start loving it and giving our best. However, if we just work for the sake of then nothing is realized and we do not remain happy in life.

We should not aim to have negative thoughts at all.

Now let's us imagine that we are not feeling at our best today, and we are having thoughts that could be classified as negative. We shouldn't be thinking such negative thoughts. We don't like the negative thoughts. **The secret of every successful man is to have, good confidence, faith and strength**

We ought to know that negative thoughts are stressful, demoralizing and depressing. We shouldn't aim to have negative thoughts at all. Often we feel uncomfortable because we think we have to say or do something in response to another person's words. When we find ourselves thinking this way, it helps enormously to take a few moments to check inside and notice what we are feeling. Negative thoughts destroy our happy livings. We ought to discard all these negative thought and act to live in a more positive atmosphere rather than living in a negative world where we can never find a happy living.

HAPPINESS LIES IN POSITIVE LIVING
BE POSITVE THINK POSITIVE LIVE POSITIVE
CHAPTER FIFTY THREE
STEPS FOR A SUCCESSFUL AND HAPPY LIFE

It might not be easy, but the positive impact it will have on our mental, emotional, and physical health will be well-worth it .At time we may think that there is no road is left for us from where we can achieve the happiness of our lives. We may also feel that life has become terrible for us to live and we are carrying new hope that someone would come to rescue us. There may be chances that someone who was there with us before might have held on to us when we were on the dark side of the life.

Life itself is a stage and we all are the performers.

What if when everything goes wrong and all the doors of happiness are closed our live becomes a silent. It is a quite common and we are aware of a marvelous proverb that Life itself is a stage and we all are the performers, performing different acts assigned to us by our almighty power. We should not forget as to what is in our possession, if it is to fulfill our duties towards our responsibility and do whatever is correct and is allowed by us in our life? We should not forget that happiness in life comes through the doors of positive thoughts; we need to have them first. If one door happen to close, another opens, in the event only when we are confident and optimistic. We have so many reasons to cry and at the same time plenty of reasons to smile as well. Similarly, happiness does not stand for anything, but is on our way of thinking that how do we keep ourselves happy in life.

Failure and disappointment are part of our life. The only thing is that we need to face and solve the problem is by keeping our dreams and hope alive be it a reason that success and happiness will come our way again.

Smiling and the doubt free character which is the foremost important reason for a successful and happy life.

There are quite a number of reasons to believe that for a successful and happy life the mystery surrounding it lies in our interests, and good memory which is the basis of our interest, power of desire and aim, keeping ourselves smiling and the doubt free character which is the foremost important reason for a successful and happy life. If we possess one solid unselfish and doubt free character within ourselves we would be quite happy and successful. The experience has taught us that we should buy some strength, hope and positivity from our loved ones to help ourselves in such a situation rather than surrendering as life is a precious gift of God and is equipped with full of joy and happiness if we help ourselves in these critical moments we can live with considerable optimism. Now let's us imagine that we are not feeling at our best today, and we are having thoughts that could be classified as negative. We shouldn't be thinking such negative thoughts. We don't like the negative thoughts. We ought to know that negative thoughts are stressful, demoralizing and depressing. We shouldn't aim to have negative thoughts at all. Often we feel uncomfortable because we think we have to say or do something in response to another person's words. When we find ourselves thinking this way, it helps enormously to take a few moments to check inside and notice what we are feeling. We are deeply depressed that negativity has governed us and has taken a deep root in our minds. So, let's imagine that you have chosen to focus on your negative thinking with regards to school.

Evaluating thoughts can generate happiness within us.

The next step is to spend a little bit of time each day evaluating your own thoughts. When you find yourself thinking critical thoughts about yourself, take a moment to pause and reflect. While you might be upset about getting a bad grade on an exam, is berating yourself really the best approach? Is there any way to put a positive spin on the situation? While you might not have done well on this exam, at least you have a better indication of how to structure your study time for the next big test. However, despite of all these good thoughts which are embodied to us by the almighty fail to revive these unwanted circumstances that lead us to sorrow and difficulties and a situation where we do not know what is correct and good for us and what is wrong for us.

Life is there, where there is hope.

We should always remember that, "Life is there, where there is hope". That single thing that remains in our hands is to find out ways to know how to overcome these worries of our life at that very moment when all doors are closed for us which means that whatever situation is there, we must not give up hope. We must fight because there have been always a chance that with good faith and hard work we can turn the odds in our favor. It is often said that it is very easy to advice but when it comes to us, things go out of our control and we fail to suggest a way out for ourselves.

Happy living allows us to tackle life's challenges

We fall into the trap of unnecessary worries and elope ourselves with negative thoughts. We feel better when somebody else is facing some difficulty but when it comes to us we fail to gather that faith, will power and the words of strength. Being a positive thinker is not about ignoring reality in favor of aspirational thoughts. It is more about taking a proactive approach to our lives. Instead of feeling hopeless or overwhelmed, positive thinking allows us to tackle life's challenges by looking for effective ways to resolve conflict and come up with creative solutions to problems. It might not be easy, but the positive impact it will have on our mental, emotional, and physical health will be well-worth it. It takes practice; lots of practice. This is not a step-by-step process that we can complete and be done with. Instead, it involves a lifelong commitment to looking inside ourselves and being willing to challenge negative thoughts and make positive changes. It is a common fact that no one in this world is free of obstacles or difficulties. If all the openings of happiness are shut for us and we have to overcome that and have no way to come out, but to survive lest we must have to learn to swim out of the sorrows because this is what is called life and sorrow free living. There are lot more examples and in many other situations, where we will find that how we could have faced and fought with our sorrows and difficulties of life when there was no hope left in our lives. As commonly said by big saints that the self- seeking man who is looking after his personal comforts and leading a lazy life for himself there would be no room for him even in the hell and he simply have lost the power of his will and he cannot lead a happy life.

The secret of every successful man is to have, good confidence

The secret of every successful man is to have, good confidence, faith and strength behind him and that remain the right cause of his single success in life. Unselfishness plays a very vital role in his life. He may not have been perfectly unselfish, yet he was tending towards it. If he had been perfectly unselfish, he would have been as great a success. The degree of unselfishness marks the degree of success everywhere and he leads to be successful man without fear worries and selfishness. Therefore creation of positivity in life is utmost necessary to enjoy the special gift of God to us. The love for God and worshipping God adds to one common thing the immense faith in Him. There may be different beliefs and ways to worship God in different communities, places and religions, but one thing remains the same and that is the Love of God for all of us. Our world is full of odds and evens, happiness and sorrows, fulfilment and emptiness. And these are all created by the Almighty. However, the most beautiful Gift of God, is Human, which is such a mystery driven by Him which could hardly be defined or explained in depth.

If aim of our life is to stay happy and let others to be happy, we will be happy and remembered by all.

We know that life cannot be foreseen. Life is not a bed of roses. Life is a battle field and not a bed of roses as every man on earth has to struggle very hard in making his life happy. But no one will actually remember us for the wealth we have gained, or success we have achieved until and unless we do not live a happy life. Life is such a special gift of Almighty and it is not gifted by Him to use it the way we like or love to. The actual path shown by Him needs to be followed by us for us to reach the peak of betterment every moment. We need to have some positive attitude to look at it comfortably but at the same time having a positive mental attitude does not mean banishing all negative thoughts and people from your life. We need to believe that a positive attitude is a choice. This step is hard to take. People are either positive or negative. They tend to blame their negativity on all kinds of outside forces fate, experiences, parents, relationship, but never really stopped to think that they could choose to be positive. Piercing ourselves that positivity is a choice has been one of the greatest things we have ever done for ourselves. Now when we find ourselves in a bad situation, we know that it's up to us to find the good, to be positive regardless of what's happening around us. We should no longer point fingers and place blame to anyone else. We need to realize that everything happens how it happens, and it's up to us to choose how we want to feel about it. We need to be in control of our attitude, and no one can take that away this from us. If we want to live a positive, joyful and happy life, we must not be surrounded by negative people who don't encourage our happiness. As a negative person, we ought to get attracted too negative people only. Only when we decide to make the change to live a more positive life, we have to get rid of our lives of the most negative influences in it. We are quite aware of the fact that no one is perfect and perfection isn't the goal when it comes to positivity but there were people in our lives who were consistently negative, who constantly bring us down, we need to stop spending so much time with them.

We can very well imagine, it is not easy for us to get away from these negative people.

It can hurt us to keep distance from people even when you know they aren't good for us and for our current lifestyle. In addition to removing negative influences from them, we also have to get rid of some of our own negative behaviors, such as the drug and alcohol abuse. We need to take some concrete steps and examine which behaviors are good for us and which were not harmful. What we need is to learn to focus on the positive things, such as working on positive activities and cultivating new, positive relationships. We must let go of the negative ones. This process may be not easy to live a positive life when negative people and behaviors continually pull us down. In every situation or in every person there is something good.

Anything good and bad is learning experience.

Most of the time it's not easy to find the positive qualities but we have to look hard to discover positivity in them. Now, when we are faced with a difficult or challenging situation, we need to think and talk to ourselves and console our mind, no matter how terrible the situation might seem, we can always find something good if we take the time to think about it. It is quite obvious that anything good and bad is learning experience so, at the very least, we must learn from bad experiences. However, there's usually even more to it than that. If you really take some time to have a look at it, we would find something good, something genuinely positive, about every person or situation. Not only do we need to be happy with ourselves for this multiple action to take effect, but we also need to be more positive and happy with others. We have to share our wealth of happiness with the people of the world. The best way is to be nice with other people, no matter what. Tell them that they look nice today. Appreciate their job and tell them that have done a great job on that assignment. Be happy and tell your elder or your kids how much you love them and how great they are. When someone is feeling down, do what we need to do is to cheer him or her up. Do send them gifts nice flower and glow them with nice notes. By doing this we will not make ourselves happy but in turn give and generate happiness for others too.At times we may suffer from chronic depression, though we know how good things look on to others life cannot be worse for us. Let's imagine how to deal when life leaves a great big steaming pile at our doorstep. Lest we need to remember that external factors can be dealt with by taking positive and happy steps to repair or at least address the root of the problem as best as we can. Whatever may be the primary cause of the problem, that cause must be examined first? What is required is that we never wanted to see the good in ourselves and, therefore, didn't want to see it in others also. We must not be critical and condescending rather we must be encouraging and supportive. We should not try to treat others as we would like to be treated, but also try to consider how we would like to be treated. The world likes to appreciate positivity, and the more we share it with others, the more we would be practicing it your own lives. When we start feeling like the idea of not being a happy person we need to remind ourselves that all it takes is one tiny step in the right direction to move towards a more happy life.

Share your happy thoughts with others

We have to believe in ourselves and remember the most important lesson of all is a happy outlook and that is a choice that we can always make. The power of remaining happy, whatever the situation, can never be underestimated. We are all here for a short duration, but is it worth it to spend any of that time in a any angry or being negative? That need to sort out in mind and soul and thus must share our happy thoughts with others. The real test of any one is to remain happy whenever some challenges become difficult. Remaining happy keeps our mind in the right state of balance and often opens resolutions to the problems at hand. Negativity is contagious and spreads like fire. It not only does its affect anyone, but it spreads to everyone who ever comes in contact with it or whoever they interact with. When only the negative perspective is in focus, the resolution process is impeded. Eliminating negativity, or rather, being positive is a mindset that can be found at any moment, and which can be turned into a habit. We must throw away the negativity in us and opt for being a very positive person this in turn will make us happy and we would be able to lead a sweet and happy life forever.

HAPPINESS LIES IN POSITIVE LIVING
BE POSITVE THINK POSITIVE LIVE POSITIVE
CHAPTER FIFTY FOUR
MAKE YOUR WAY TO HAPPY LIVING

We need to learn a lesson from every situation. No matter how difficult the situation may appear. We should recognize the beautiful lessons waiting to be discovered. Sometimes lessons may prove to be expensive and costly, but every problem is a learning experience in disguise. We need to be conscious of our thoughts, especially, when life just isn't going our way. The moment we see that we are diving into frustration, agony, sorrow or low self –esteem we must shift our thoughts, by thinking about something completely different and unrelated. You are essentially trying to cultivate a new habit here, the secret of successful and happy life lies in keeping ourselves smiling and the character which is the foremost important reason that lies within us. Whenever your mind is tempted to jump the fence and start to worry, say this verse aloud or to yourself. You may even have to repeat it over and over again. Am I constantly striving to see the positive in every aspect of my life? Steps for a successful and happy life.

MAKE YOUR WAY TO HAPPY LIVING

We need to believe that a happy living is a matter of our choice. This step is hard to take. People are either positive or negative. They tend to blame their negativity on all kinds of outside forces fate, experiences, parents, relationship, but never really stopped to think that they could choose to be happy. Piercing ourselves that happiness is a choice has been one of the greatest things we have ever done for ourselves. Now when we find ourselves in a bad situation, we know that it is up to us to find the good, to be happy regardless of what is happening around us. We should no longer point fingers and place blame to anyone else. We need to realise that everything happens how it happens, and it is up to us to choose how we want to feel about it. We need to be in control of our attitude and happiness, and no one can take that away this from us.

Unhappiness is contagious and spreads like fire.

It not only does its affect anyone, but it spreads to everyone who ever comes in contact with it or whoever they interact with. When only the negative perspective is in focus, the resolution process is impeded. Eliminating unhappiness, or rather, being happy is a mindset that can be found at any moment, and which can be turned into a habit. If we want to live a happy, joyful life, we must not be surrounded by negative people who don't encourage our happiness. As a negative person, we ought to get attracted to negative people only. Only when we decide to make the change to live a more positive and happy life, we have to get rid of our lives of the most negative influences in it. We are quite aware of the fact that no one is perfect and perfection is not the goal when it comes to positivity but there were people in our lives who were consistently negative, who constantly bring us down, we need to stop spending so much time with them. We can very well imagine, it is not easy for us to get away from these unhappy people. It can hurt us to keep distance from people even when you know they are not good for us and for our current lifestyle. In addition to removing negative influences from them, we also have to get rid of some of our own negative behaviors, such as the drug and alcohol abuse. We need to take some concrete steps and examine which behaviors are good for us and which were not harmful. What we need is to learn to focus on the happy things, such as working on positive activities and cultivating new, positive relationships. We must let go of the negative ones. This process may be not easy to live a positive life when negative people and behaviors continually pull us down. We need to discard all of them to lead a happy and sweet life. An art of sweet living lies below us we have only to recognize it. The real test of any one is to remain happy whenever some challenges become difficult. Remaining happy keeps our mind in the right state of balance and often opens resolutions to the problems at hand. We must throw away the unhappiness in us and opt for being a very positive person. In every situation or in every person there is something good. Most of the time it's not easy to find the happiness qualities but we have to look hard to discover happiness in them.

The secret of successful and happy life lies in keeping ourselves smiling

Now, when we are faced with a difficult or challenging situation, we need to think and talk to ourselves and console our mind, no matter how terrible the situation might seem, we can always find something good if we take the time to think about it. It is quite obvious that anything good and bad is learning experience so, at the very least, we must learn from bad experiences. However, there is usually even more to it than that. If you really take some time to have a look at it, we would find something good, something genuinely happy, about every person or situation. We must look for sweet living in life

Get Sweet feeling in your life

Once we start thinking more in a happy manner, we will realize that we had to reinforce these thoughts and behaviors within ourselves so that we could stick to it. As with any sort of training, the more we practice, the better we get to be happy. The best and easiest way to do this is to be happy when it comes to who we are. We need to speak to ourselves that we are awesome. And we have done a good job at work thus creating happiness within us. We need to be honest with ourselves, and we need to do our best to look for the good. And, whatever we do, we must not focus on the negative. It is alright not to like everything about ourselves, but don not focus on what we do not like. We have all to get the sweet feeling in our lives, and it is up to us to remind ourselves of them every day.Not only do we need to be happy with ourselves for this multiple action to take effect, but we need to be more happy with others too. We have to share our wealth of happiness with the people of the world. The best way is to be nice with other people and to make them happy, no matter what the matter is. Tell them that they look nice today.

Share sweet and happy thoughts

What is required is that we never wanted to see the good in ourselves and, therefore, didn't want to see it in others also. We must not be critical and condescending rather we must be encouraging and supportive. We should not try to treat others as we would like to be treated, but also try to consider how we would like to be treated. This will strangle the pattern of self-pity, mind-created imaginations, and negative downward stairs. Really what makes us different from other mammals is our ability to control our thoughts and think for ourselves happiness and shift our unhappy thoughts to a happy feelings and to happy living. We may have made mistakes, but now we can accept it and continue, knowing that we will make a different decision in the future. If we understand this it can be appreciative for the experience. We cannot be both angry and grateful at the same time. We should start counting the blessings and miracles in our lives and if we start exploring for them and we would find more happiness in doing so.

Feeling good about ourselves and showing self-confidence.

Feeling good about ourselves and showing self-confidence boosts our skills potential and capabilities in any areas of work and supports us to become happier. We need to shift our thoughts from being a unhappy person to more strong and positive man. Also keeping in mind that pushing things to the limit and going beyond what we think is possible for us to get to the next step of being happy. It becomes another key to achieving what we really want to do. We only want happiness and want to lead a happy life.Even if it may even be relationships and we are finding it difficult to meet someone where we are actually interested in, we need not wait because it usually doesn't come to us by own, we must stand up to get help from any learned fellow One of the most important things while doing all of this is to be happy about what we are doing, thus we ought to have a successful goal setting our lifestyle with a happy attitude. We may or may not be able to solve the problem of unhappiness that lies within us, but at least knowing that we are taking positive steps that can help us improve our happiness. It will not be easy, of course, for us and it may be like suffering a chronic disease thus we must balance ourselves as "being happy" with an understanding that the reality is, it is going to be an ongoing battle for our own survival. Depression will undermine even the strongest of wills, need help to maintain or at least be reminded of a happy outlook and happiness that is prevailing within us.Counseling, psychotherapy, and the right combination of medication will play a crucial role in helping to keep us from sinking into that very dark place that is the essence of depression and unhappiness. Be patient, but don't look for miracles. It may be that we will need the help of professionals throughout our lives to maintain a generally even keel. If one could "will away" depression, there would be no need of doctors or drugs. What we can do is understand why we feel like we do, and explain to our counselors that we wish it were that easy, and that we appreciate our concern towards being happy persons. Shifting our thoughts enables us to the right path of our happiness and thinking in its direction of positivity can make us to lead a very happy life.

HAPPINESS LIES IN POSITIVE LIVING

BE POSITVE THINK POSITIVE LIVE POSITIVE

CHAPTER FIFTY FIVE

LEAD A TENSION FREE AND HAPPY LIFE

It is often said that mindfulness meditation helps people to develop the skill of being detached and aware. As a result we can become aware of these core irrational beliefs about self, others, and the world without activating self-destructive survival behaviors driven by high stress. We ought to know the simple ways to get people into using mindfulness meditation.. A little stress to keep us energized motivated and hanging out with the people that are doing healthy things. Having a stable relationship these all the primarily things we ought to gather within ourselves. We have to be on the lookout for a possible date with someone. We may even join special groups or clubs of people within our age bracket and who share the same interest. Join church events as well. Try new activities. By expanding our horizon, we will get to know more people who can be a potential date of having a good company.   Let us keep life simple. Many of us are always over looking for the most complicated way of doing things in life. We can make our lives to be more simple just take a walk through the park, or a quiet evening with the family. We need not clutter our lives with unnecessary decisions by making everything complicated and complex why not try to keep it simple. Why not practice to be satisfied. Many people don't know how to be satisfied with what life gives them. They are so busy wanting more that they squander what life has already given them. Always urging for more and demanding to have everything making themselves and lives more complicated. Why not practice to be more satisfied we need most. What we need to beware is of indecision. Life is not that easy at times we have to make tough choices. Never put off a decision that we can make on the day. At times we may miss some of the best and most exciting opportunities in the world because we were indecisive. People who are successful people do not fall prey back and forth on decisions. Let us practice cheerfulness and be happy We have heard it several times before, and we would hear it here again and again – it only takes a few seconds to smile! We need not be surprised as to how well being cheerful to others can spread like wildfire and make us happy. We live in a society where often glumness is the ruled. A simple smile or kind word can spread through our culture like a fire – not only will we feel better, but those who interact with us will also feel better and best. Therefore why we should not practice cheerfulness and make ourselves happy. How about if we learn to like people and make ourselves happy. We don't have to love everyone we meet; we simply need to learn to like people – especially those who are different than us. Often we may not agree with everything what they do, or maybe with all of their beliefs, but by learning to get along with them we will open our mind up to change – a critical trait that is absolutely necessary in world of today. The most important thing that we must learn is to Live and let live. Is it really our concern what the guy across the other lane wants to do something with his life or wants to share his life with? Why not we learn to live our lives to the fullest and let others live their life to their fullest. We need to bear in mind that we are not above anyone else, and none of us should think we should be allowed to dictate how another person should live and lead their lives. Stop beating over the past happening and let us forgive ourselves. It is simple let us stop beating things that happened in the past – things what we have done or we did not do, and the awful mistakes that we may have made. Forgiving oneself is a unique skill and only few of us have the ability to accomplish. It's such a shame that we spent a lifetime living in the past and never make it to our full potential in the future. We must forgive ourselves and just as importantly, forgive others too. It may seem to be a difficult task but if we encourage each other and stop beating over the past we will live a more meaningful, happy and fulfilled life.

HAPPINESS LIES IN POSITIVE LIVINGBE

POSITVE THINK POSITIVE LIVE POSITIVE

CHAPTER FIFTY SIX

BRING BACK YOUR LIFE TO NORMAL

We need to remember that as we possibly as we can we should make it a point to eat a more balanced, and healthy diet even though we may very little money left with us. We have intake of lot of greens vegetables and with variety of fruit and nuts which are all super healthy food for us, and which are less expensive than meats, cheeses, and processed foods! Their nitrifying value will energize and elevate our body, and knowing this that we are treating ourselves will surely refresh our minds. If we look for rich food rich in vitamins and other useful ingredients which include nuts, soya beans and fatty fish we would get more nutrition value. We must cut back on the caffeine drinks, alcohol. We don't have to quit, but reducing the intake of them will help reduce anxiety and stress from time to time. Exercise is one of health sport that our body needs most. It may be yoga, cross training, or even a simple walking in the park. This helps keeping our body active and will also help to grow our outlook. If we make it hobby we would enjoy the most. Whether its art, photography, music focusing on something other than the worry factor it will give our mind some good atmosphere to breathe off and would generate a good behavior within us. The other refreshing factor is naturally our sleep. We need not be reminded of this. Our body is probably begging us for it when we are in the middle of hard times. We may be drawn to maintain good sleeping habits. Maintain a consistent sleep schedule, but allow yourself some leeway. If we sleep peacefully let our body get about 8 hours of sleep we get the best results. If you're just starting to have those thoughts, speak to your physician or your therapist. They may prescribe something to help steer you back to the center, emotionally. It may be the act of talking about it is therapeutic enough, but don't assume that. Leave that call to the professionals. Having goals which are set again and again after each one is achieved will give you a mindset or target to strive for which leads to success, with success becomes natural positive attitude. With all costiveness, goals and success builds a higher potential and belief within yourself. Setting realistic goals that you know you can achieve by staying positive is a great beginning to success. Your attitude around your friends, family and public people really tells them who you are, being positive instead of negative makes an excellent first impression on anybody. Positive means to be absolute, clear-cut, definite, forward-looking and expressively firm with a decision. Having a positive attitude toward something means you are willing to commit and do the work without complaint, which leads to goals. You realize that what appears negative today will change tomorrow. Nothing stays the same. Whether you are positive or negative, the situation does not change. So, we mind as well be positive. As with any habit, the habit of remaining positive in all situations takes practice and a commitment to yourself to take control. But start small, start paying attention to your emotions, start by wanting to change. Don't hold onto anything that bothers your mind. It can only hurt your health and it won't help your problems at all. The people that live the longest in this world do not hold grudges or hold onto negative feelings. Visualize your worries on a large chalkboard in your mind. Watch yourself take a big eraser and erase the problems. Every time the thoughts come back into your head, see yourself with the eraser again. Therefore do not worry about tomorrow, for tomorrow will worry about itself. Each day has enough trouble of its own. Do not anticipate trouble, or worry about what may never happen. Keep in the sunlight. Imagine every day to be the last of a life surrounded with hopes, cares, anger and fear. The hours that come unexpectedly will be much the more grateful. The mind that is anxious about future events is miserable. Present fears are less than horrible imaginings. Let us be of good cheer, remembering that the misfortunes hardest to bear are those that never happen, focus on the positive aspects of their lives, rather than on the negative setbacks. "Feeling confident affects the way we perceive our situations and how we decide to manage them. Don't waste your life in doubts and fears: spend yourself on the work before you, well assured that the right performance of this hour's duties will be the best preparation for the hours or ages that follow it. It is not work that kills men, it is worry. Work is healthy; you can hardly put more on a man than he can bear. But worry is rust upon the blade. It is not movement that destroys the machinery, but friction. Never let life's hardships disturb you ... no one can avoid problems, not even saints or sages. As with any habit, the habit of remaining positive in all situations takes practice and a commitment to yourself to take control. Life is what you make it, so make it a happy one!! Don't worry on things that may not happen, life is to short to worry to much. Smile and be happy. Focus your imagination and make efforts on becoming new positive person. Create happiness in you. Divert your mind to good thoughts. It is much easier to bring about change if you just put your mind to it and change your thoughts into a much more positive direction. We know that it is difficult for us to control things that happen in our lives, but we can, with some effort, control what we think or do in our lives. Positive thoughts will make our imagination livelier and we would be able to lead our lives happily without many worries.

The second good step is to have the company of good and positive living friends.

Appreciate the people in your life who have stood by you through thick and thin. Count their support and analyses the happiness in them which will help you to lead a much happier life. Good friends help each other in the days of crises and through both the good and bad times. Keep yourself busy and surround yourself with good friends, who always think positive.

Feel positive about them and feel lucky to have them in your company. Share positive thoughts with them. Tell them to be happy and to lead a sweet good and happy life.

The third step is to focus your imagination on happy things in life by giving a good smile.

The easiest way is feeling happy. Many theories have revealed that happiness can lift one's mood and can divert your mind to sweet living. We may also share positivity with others by flashing them with a brilliant and good smile. Positive and sweet talks are the rewards of good and happy thoughts it generates more happiness. Dejection, disappointments and depression, however, have consequences that could ruin our health, and life. We must divert their minds to focus to the imagination of good and happy life. If something bad or good is to happen it is sure to happen, whether we are sad or unhappy or depressed. Let us put our energy into today and stop worrying about the future and past. We should not foresee trouble, or worry about what may never happen as past is dead and gone forever and future is uncertain and yet to come. Be your unabashed self in all the best ways that you can.

The basic facts we should know about happiness.

The basic techniques to analyze happiness and how to break the unhappy habits before it breaks us. These are the simple ways where we can concentrate and get rid of unhappy thoughts. Annalise unhappiness to see and get the reasons and facts as to why we worry. To avoid reoccurrence of worries, concentrate on prayers as prayers are the best source of remedies of the prevailing worries. The more you pray, the less you'll panic. The more you worship, the less you worry. There is nothing that wastes the body like worry, and anyone who has any faith in God should need not to worry about anything whatsoever is to happen in future. This will ease our way to a sweet good and happy living.

What do we think about happy thoughts?

The feeling of happiness is within us. It is said that sweet good and happy living is purely our own matter and it has nothing to do with our external circumstances. There is something very special within us which keeps us happy and there is something very unpleasant within us which keeps unhappy. Yes quite true it is the positiveness within us that make and creates happiness within us. Happy living through positivity is nothing more than that of living a normal life free from undue pressures, problems and tensions. If we want to live a happy life then we need to get rid of the negativity and we must try to avoid all the unpleasant things within us which makes us unhappy.

Negative approach always complicates the problems and increases unhappiness.

Most of us do the fatal mistake of looking outwards for happiness rather than looking inwards. Be happy, be strong, be bold and be courageous every day. Even if we are having a bad day, think of some good things that may come our way, either later that day, tomorrow, next week, month, or next moment.

Simply making castles in the air won't solve our problems.

When everything seems to be beyond our control, it's almost too easy for us to slip into the grasp of unhappiness. To avoid unhappiness we must strive to abolish this sort of thinking through the power of thinking positively. We ought to know the basic fundamental of analyzing happiness. Worries and unhappiness create unnecessary thoughts and these are caused by people going in for unwanted decisions, fore hand not even knowing as to when a good decision is made and not even having sufficient knowledge about it. We must first study and after carefully weighing all the facts than only come to a powerful decision. Simply making castles in the air won't solve our problems but add more to our vows and unhappiness which may even lead us to unhappy life. Anxiety and worry can go hand in hand. When anxiety grabs the mind, it is self-perpetuating. Your mind gets clogged with numerous buts and ifs. Do not worry about your life.

Negativity and worries are repetitive thoughts

Negativity and worries are repetitive thoughts associated with feelings of anxiety in anticipation of some negative future event. Worries and anxious feelings lead to disasters and make our lives unhappy. If we know that our circumstances are beyond our control or power we need to change them or revise them to our liking. We must try to put a stop-less order on our worries. We must be careful and we need not permit little things which become insects of our lives to ruin our happiness. Co-operate with the inevitable. Decide just how much anxiety a thing may be worth and refuse to give in anymore. All the happiness is not given in one go it comes slowly and slowly. We must pay special attention to remain happy and be happy. Keep ourselves happy, treat our worried thoughts as valuable signals to a sweet living good and happy living.

The utmost cause of unhappiness is your state of depression. Unhappiness is not there to motivate information gathering or problem-solving. In fact it is depression that constructs the future of unhappiness. Depression is inertia. That's the thing about depression: depression is so insidious, and it compounds daily, and it's impossible to ever see the end of it.

Keep yourself happy

Depressed people think they know themselves, but maybe they only know depression. There are no hopeless than this to get depressed create unhappiness in our minds and become unhappy all the time. Our attitude towards suffering and depression becomes very important because it can affect how we cope with suffering when it arises. Depression is nourished by a lifetime of grieved and unforgiven causes. Another factor to remain unhappy is worrying about unwanted and useless things. Worry is a misuse of the imagination. To keep yourself happy, treat your worried thoughts as most unwanted assets. These are the fundamental facts you should be familiar about worries. A huge factor to stay happy is to cater your worries around, an important relationship in your life and pay special attention sustaining positive relationships. Make your mind firm and do come to a positive decision and not allow the worries to un-ease the power your mind and soul that can cause unhappiness in you.

We must free ourselves from fruitless worry.

Once a decision is carefully reached we should get busy carrying out our decisions and should not bother about all the anxieties that are about to come. When we, or any of our colleagues or associates, are about to worry about a problem, we must write it out and think of the following questions: Instead of worrying about what people say, why not spend time trying to accomplish something they may admire. What if we just acted like everything was easy? How would your life be different if we stopped worrying about things we can't control and started focusing on the things we can? Let today be the day. We must free ourselves from fruitless worry, seize the day and take effective action on things we can change thus we would see that our lives changes for the betterment and we are on the right path of a sweet, good and happy living.

HAPPINESS LIES IN POSITIVE LIVING
BE POSITVE THINK POSITIVE LIVE POSITIVE
CHAPTER FIFTY SEVEN

BRING BACK YOUR HAPPY DAYS

We need to remember that as we possibly as we can we should make it a point to eat a more balanced, and healthy diet even though we may very little money left with us. We have intake of lot of greens vegetables and with variety of fruit and nuts which are all super healthy food for us, and which are less expensive than meats, cheeses, and processed foods! Their nitrifying value will energize and elevate our body, and knowing this that we are treating ourselves will surely refresh our minds. If we look for rich food rich in vitamins and other useful ingredients which include nuts, soya beans and fatty fish we would get more nutrition value. We must cut back on the caffeine drinks, alcohol. We don't have to quit, but reducing the intake of them will help reduce anxiety and stress from time to time.Exercise is one of health sport that our body needs most. It may be yoga, cross training, or even a simple walking in the park. This helps keeping our body active and will also help to grow our outlook. If we make it hobby we would enjoy the most. Whether its art, photography, music focusing on something other than the worry factor it will give our mind some good atmosphere to breathe off and would generate a good behavior within us. The other refreshing factor is naturally our sleep. We need not be reminded of this. Our body is probably begging us for it when we are in the middle of hard times. We may be drawn to maintain good sleeping habits. Maintain a consistent sleep schedule, but allow yourself some leeway. If we sleep peacefully let our body get about 8 hours of sleep we get the best results. If you're just starting to have those thoughts, speak to your physician or your therapist. They may prescribe something to help steer you back to the center, emotionally. It may be the act of talking about it is therapeutic enough, but don't assume that. Leave that call to the professionals. Having goals which are set again and again after each one is achieved will give you a mindset or target to strive for which leads to success, with success becomes natural positive attitude. With all costiveness, goals and success builds a higher potential and belief within yourself. Setting realistic goals that you know you can achieve by staying positive is a great beginning to success. Your attitude around your friends, family and public people really tells them who you are, being positive instead of negative makes an excellent first impression on anybody. Positive means to be absolute, clear-cut, definite, forward-looking and expressively firm with a decision. Having a positive attitude toward something means you are willing to commit and do the work without complaint, which leads to goals. You realize that what appears negative today will change tomorrow. Nothing stays the same. Whether you are positive or negative, the situation does not change. So, we mind as well be positive. As with any habit, the habit of remaining positive in all situations takes practice and a commitment to yourself to take control. But start small, start paying attention to your emotions, start by wanting to change. Don't hold onto anything that bothers your mind. It can only hurt your health and it won't help your problems at all. The people that live the longest in this world do not hold grudges or hold onto negative feelings. Visualize your worries on a large chalkboard in your mind. Watch yourself take a big eraser and erase the problems. Every time the thoughts come back into your head, see yourself with the eraser again. Therefore do not worry about tomorrow, for tomorrow will worry about itself. Each day has enough trouble of its own. Do not anticipate trouble, or worry about what may never happen. Keep in the sunlight. Imagine every day to be the last of a life surrounded with hopes, cares, anger and fear. The hours that come unexpectedly will be much the more grateful. The mind that is anxious about future events is miserable. Present fears are less than horrible imaginings. Let us be of good cheer, remembering that the misfortunes hardest to bear are those that never happen, focus on the positive aspects of their lives, rather than on the negative setbacks. "Feeling confident affects the way we perceive our situations and how we decide to manage them. Don't waste your life in doubts and fears: spend yourself on the work before you, well assured that the right performance of this hour's duties will be the best preparation for the hours or ages that follow it. It is not work that kills men, it is worry. Work is healthy; you can hardly put more on a man than he can bear. But worry is rust upon the blade. It is not movement that destroys the machinery, but friction. Never let life's hardships disturb you ... no one can avoid problems, not even saints or sages. As with any habit, the habit of remaining positive in all situations takes practice and a commitment to yourself to take control. Life is what you make it, so make it a happy one!! Don't worry on things that may not happen, life is to short to worry to much. Smile and be happy

HAPPINESS LIES IN POSITIVE LIVING
BE POSITVE THINK POSITIVE LIVE POSITIVE

CHAPTER FIFTY EIGHT

OUR OTHER PUBLICATION

ARE ON SALE

"MICROSCOPY OF ASTROLOGY"

"MICROSCOPY OF NUMEROLOGY"

"MICROSCOPY OF REMEDIES"

MICROSCOPY OF HAPPY LIVING

MICROSCOPY OF TRANSITING PLANETS

HAPPINESS LIES IN POSITIVE LIVING

BE POSITVE THINK POSITIVE LIVE POSITIVE

CHAPTER FIFTY NINE

OUR CONTACT ADDRESS:

PLEASE SEND YOUR QUERIES TO:

BALDEV BHATIA

CONSULTANT-NUMEROLOGY-ASTROLOGY

C-63, FIRST FLOOR

MALVIYA NAGAR

NEW DELHI-110017

INDIA

TEL NO 919810075249

TEL NO 91 11 26686856

TEL NO 91 7503280786

TEL NO 91 7702735880

HAPPINESS LIES IN POSITIVE LIVING

BE POSITVE THINK POSITIVE LIVE POSITIVE

CHAPTER SIXTY

OUR MOST SOUGHT WEB SITES:

HTTP://WWW.ASTROLOGYBB.COM

HTTP://WWW.BBASTROLOGY.COM

HTTP://WWW.BALDEVBHATIA.COM

HTTP://WWW.BALDEVBHATIA.US

HTTP://WWW.BALDEVBHATIA.ORG

HTTP://WWW.BALDEVBHATIA.INFO

HTTP://WWW.BALDEVBHATIA.NET

HTTP://WWW.BALDEVBHATIA.BIZ

HTTP://WWW.BALDEVBHATIA.IN

HAPPINESS LIES IN POSITIVE LIVING

BE POSITVE THINK POSITIVE LIVE POSITIVE

CHAPTER SIXTY ONE

SPECIAL NOTE

FROM THE AUTHOR BALDEV BHATIA

THANK YOU FOR READING MY BOOK

MY SINCERE PRAYERS

FOR ALL MY READERS

"GOD BLESS YOU ALL"

"ANY ONE WHO READS AND KEEPS THIS BOOK AS HOLY MANUSCRIPT, GOD IS SURE TO BLESS HIM, WITH ALL THE PEACE, HAPPINESS, WEALTH, HEALTH AND PROSPERITY OF THIS UNIVERSE"

BALDEV BHATIA

www.ingramcontent.com/pod-product-compliance
Lightning Source LLC
Chambersburg PA
CBHW071328280526
45787CB00001B/25